Enhancing Mental Wellness in Adolescents:
The Power of Spirituality, Resilience, and Personality

Neha Singh

CONTENTS

ABBREVIATIONS

S.I.	Spiritual Intelligence
C.E.T.	Critical Existence Thinking
P.M.P.	Personal Meaning Production
T.A.	Transcendent Awareness
C.S.E.	Conscious State Expansion
Support GMSR	Giving and Maintaining Supportive Relationship
Support HUSR	Having and Using Supportive Relationships
M.H.	Mental Health

LIST OF TABLES

PREFACE

The adolescent stage of human development is the final stage of childhood, after which the person is generally accepted as an adult human being, period of major changes, both physiological as well as psychological. This phase is also considered as an important educational transition point when the adolescent seeks to establish an identity for himself through achievement of academic and career goals. The individual is expected to navigate through demanding situations and tough challenges to uncover the endless possibilities that adolescence brings. In doing so, many individuals succumb to pressure while some show remarkable persistence to eventually attain competence. This phenomenon of achieving favourable outcomes despite adversity is known as resilience. Spiritual intelligence is the capacity of an individual to possess a socially relevant purpose in life by understanding self and having a high degree of conscience, compassion, and commitment to human values. Human values are effective in people's physical and mental health whereas personality is the dynamic organization within the individual of that psychophysical system which determines his unique adjustments to the environment, his life and values, holiness feeling in life, the more balanced perception of values and believing to the improvement of the world.

Although the topic of spiritual intelligence, resilience, and personality has been at the center of much attention in the past couple of decades, most investigation in India focused on spiritual intelligence, resilience, personality and mental health in the aftermath of disasters. Additionally research conducted in the area is to see the role of spiritual intelligence, resilience and personality together on the mental health of adolescents. Hence, there still remains a dearth of studies investigating spiritual intelligence, resilience and mental health among adolescents in our cultural context. Besides, there is a direction necessary for measuring in Indian context.

The present investigation is an attempt to examine the role of spiritual intelligence, resilience and personality in the mental health of adolescents of 17-19 years of age group. Besides, it also attempts to answer whether these variables predict the mental health of adolescents. This study also assesses that individual with high spiritual intelligence and resilience show better mental health. Finally, the relationship between spiritual intelligence, resilience, personality and mental health outcome was also determined.

The thesis is divided into six chapters. Chapter I deals with the introduction to the relevant concept of the study. Chapter II presents a review of available literature, along with rationale, objectives and hypotheses framed for the study. Chapter III outlines the research design, tool, and methodology used in this research. In Chapter IV, the results have been presented in the light of prior investigations. Chapter V deals with discussion of the study. Finally, VI presents a summary of the work and the conclusion derived from it.

CHAPTER- I

INTRODUCTION

The word adolescence is derived from the latin word 'adolescere' which means to grow into maturity. Adolescence is a complex stage of life and a critical period of biological and physiological changes, characterized by accelerated growth and development. (Carr-Gregg & Shale 2002; Takanishi 1993; Mwamwenda 1996; Adams & Berzonsky 2003; Balk 1995 Burt 2002 and Williams & Mc Gillicuddy-De Lisi 2000).

It is the stage of rapid change of an individual's physical, mental, social, moral and spiritual outlook. The adolescent experiences change both internally and externally. The internal changes include biological and physiological changes which are age-related. External changes include environmental demands and expectation that family and society place on them during the time of cognitive development and maturation.

Adolescents are expected to cope with these internal and external changes and to adapt to their new roles in society and the family. These rapid changes in development may cause adaptation problems and affect adolescent's mental health. In this period foundation for future education, major life roles, relationships, and working towards long-term goals are established. Adolescence as a formative stage plays a significant role in the study of developmental psychopathology because, after this maturational interval, it is difficult to change some behavioural and emotional patterns. Thus, this period is the very important period of life as it lays the foundation for the future of an individual. Literature reflects that numerous studies have focused on various factors for increasing individual's mental health (Buss, 2000; Lyubomirsky, 2001).

As the adolescents are experiencing numerous robust cognitive and physical changes for the first time in their lives, they begin to look at their friends, their generation as additional vital and influential than their parents. Due to peer pressure, they generally indulge in activities not deemed socially acceptable, though this might be more of a social phenomenon than a psychological one. This overlap is addressed within the study of psycho-sociology.

The family is an important factor of adolescent's psychology. Family environment and family have a substantial impact on the developing minds of teenagers and these developments may reach a climax during adolescence. For example, abusive parents may lead a child to "poke fun" at other classmates when he/she is seven years old or so, but during adolescence, it might worsen progressively. If the concepts and theory behind right and wrong were not established early in child's life, the lack of this knowledge may impaired a teenager's ability to make useful decisions as well as allowing his/her impulses to control his/her decisions.

In the exploration for a unique social identity for themselves, adolescents are frequently confused about "right" and "wrong". G. Stanley Hall (1904) denoted this era as "storms and stresses". Consistent with him, conflict at this developmental stage is normal and not unusual. Mead (1928), on the other hand, attributed the behavior of adolescents to their culture and upbringing. However, Piaget attributed this stage in development with greatly increased cognitive abilities; at this stage of life the individual's thoughts begin taking a lot of an abstract type and the egocentric thoughts decrease, hence the individual is able to think in a wider perspective.

Spiritual Intelligence

The concept of spiritual intelligence relies on spirituality. The term spiritual intelligence was coined by Zohar (1997) and it is derived from Latin word 'wind or Breath'. Literally, this term means the wind that is blowing through us, the principle that makes us alive and human. Spiritual intelligence forms the part of our total intelligence. The word 'spiritual' proposes images of scared experiences and personal reality and the soul as the subjective and personal reality. The word 'intelligence' stands for 'mind at work' analytic problem-solving.

According to Zohar (2000) "spiritual intelligence is access to the use of meaning, vision and value in the way that we think and the decision that we make". It is the intelligence that creates us whole and also provides us with our integrity. It is the soul's Intelligence, the intelligence of deep self that with that tend to raise the fundamental question and with that tend to we reframe our answer.

Some of the underlying principles of Spiritual intelligence given by Zohar (2003) are as follows:

- Knowing ourselves, our beliefs, value and what really motivates us i.e., self-awareness.
- Deep gratitude for everything we have received in life and everyone who has helped us.
- An ability to forgive others who have hurt us and ability to apologizes when we hurt others.
- The ability to be flexible and spontaneous-to adapt and react to a reality which changes from moment to moment.
- The virtue of being inspired by the vision and value-letting our vision lead us and acting in accordance with our principle and values.
- Being able to see larger pattern, relationship and the connection between things, a sense of belonging to humanity, the community of life and the entire universe i.e. holism.
- Compassion
- To respect and value other people and life forms for their differences.
- A tendency to "field independence": standing up for one's own conviction and
- Being able to go against the world.

Spiritual intelligence is occupied with the inner life of mind and spirit and its relationship to being in the world. It implies a capacity for a deep understanding of existential question and sight into multiple levels of consciousness. It is more than individual's mental ability. Spiritual Intelligence illuminates the mind, inspires the soul and opens the hearts, connecting the individual's human psyche to the underlying ground of being. It can be developed with practice and can help a person to distinguish reality from illusion. It may be expressed in any culture as love, wisdom, and service. Spiritual intelligence includes various methods that can coordinate innate life and spiritual with the extent of life and it may lead to well-being and importance of life quality (Vaughan, 2003).Wigglesworth (2002) conceived spiritual intelligence as the ability to behave with compassion and wisdom while maintaining inner and outer peace regardless of the circumstances. Thus it can be said that spiritual intelligence is the consequence of the highest level of individual growth in the fields of cognition, meaning attainment, transcendental and moral communication (Vaughan, 2002). It involves an array of capabilities derived from a spiritual resource in line with the advancement of an emotional intelligence construct.

Spiritual intelligence is effective in people's physical and mental health. It includes having the feeling of meaning and mission toward lives and values, holiness feeling in life, the more balanced perception of values and believing to the improvement of the world. This intelligence is a set of capabilities, capacities, and a spiritual resource which leads to adaptability and consequently people's mental health (King, 2008; Zohar and Marshall, 2000).

Psychologists have tried to give their views working in their area. Robert Emmons (2000) further conceptualizes spiritual intelligence as the adaptive use of spiritual information to facilitate everyday problem solving and goal attainment. According to Zohar and Marshall (2004) spiritual intelligence is a tool through which we assess our deepest meaning, values, purpose and highest motivation.

Wolman (2001) also demonstrated spiritual intelligence as " human capacity to ask ultimate question about the meaning of life and to simultaneously experience the seamless connection between each of us and the world in which we live".

Vaughan (2002) regarded spiritual intelligence as a power to a profound understanding of existing question and perception about various awareness levels and the awareness of individual relationship to the earth and all forms of life. He has identified three components of spiritual intelligence i.e., power to form a meaning that is rooted on a profound knowledge of existential question, responsiveness in the utilization of multiple consciousness levels aimed to properly address the problem and, attentiveness regarding the interconnection of each individual as well as to the transcendent.

Similarly, Nasel (2004) defined spiritual intelligence as the capacity in bringing out one spiritual gifts and resources for further recognition search for meaning, and the resolution to certain existential spiritual and practical matter. These resources and potentialities could be a prayer, intuition or transcendence which is correlated in simplifying the abilities to seek for meaning of one's existence facilitation of solving issues, and the improving one's power for adaptive decision making.

Robert Emmons (2004) further conceptualized spiritual intelligence as the adaptive use of intelligence, use of spiritual information to facilitate everyday problem solving and goal attainment. Zohar and Marshall (2004) have also portrayed spiritual intelligence as a tool through which we access our deepest meaning, values, purposes and highest motivation.

Smith (2005) concluded that spiritual intelligence is incidental to the better adaptation with environment and the more intelligent; the more pressure could be endured. According to Smith (2005) some underlying principles of spirituality are: (i) spiritual experience; having special spiritual experience and activities; (ii) stress suppression; enjoying faith and religious belief in order to solve problems; (iii) objective: regarding religious issues in order to have special objective: (iv) Living out: keeping distance from stereotyped beliefs; (v) beliefs centrality: influence of religious on the behavior and performance (e.g. eating, drinking, wearing); (vi) religious practice: saying prayers and doing religious actions; (vii) endurance: accepting the beliefs of other religions, (ix) religious concepts: believing in religious.

In another definition George (2006) states that spiritual intelligence assists in finding the deepest and most inner resources from an individual from which the capacity to care, the power to tolerate and adaptation is obtained.

Arman regarded (2009), spiritual intelligence as a kind of ability that causes self-consciousness, self control, profound understanding of meaning of life, purposefulness, increase in peace, the ability to communicate effectively with others and mental health. According to him spiritual intelligence comprises seven major components viz., **consciousness** which means growth of advanced awareness and self-knowledge that brings out innate translogical knowing, attentive, attentive and spiritual practices; **grace** means to live in accordance with the scared with the manifestation of trust and love about life that is rooted from happiness, beauty and gratefulness; **meaning** refers encountering the importance of everyday endeavor through a sense of purpose and a need for service embracing the presence of pain and suffering; **transcendent** is running away from self-worth into interrelated wholeness covering a holistic system standpoint and fostering the human relationship by understanding, sympathy and orientation; **peaceful** surrender means peacefully submitting to higher self (god, truth, absolute, or true nature) that includes self completeness, self-acceptance, calmness, humbleness and egolessness; and **inner directedness** means an innate free will in line with accountable and sensible action involving judgment truthfulness and freedom from attachment, conditioning and anxiousness.

In another definition King (2008) has determined spiritual intelligence as a set of adaptive mental capacities based on non-material and transcendent self and mastery of spiritual states. King further suggests four core abilities/capacities of spiritual intelligence. Firstly, **critical existential thinking** which means the capacity to critically contemplate the nature of existence, reality, the universe, space, time, and other existential / metaphysical issues; also the ability to contemplate non-existential issues in relation to one's existence (i.e., from existential perspective). Secondly, **perspective meaning production** means the ability to derive personal meaning and purpose from all physical and mental experiences, including the capacity to create and master a life purpose. Thirdly, **transcendental awareness** is the capacity to identify transcendent dimension patterns of the self (i.e., a transpersonal or transcendent self), of others, and of the physical world (e.g.; not materialism) during normal states of consciousness, accompanied by the capacity to their relationship to one's self and to the physical. Fourthly, **conscious state expansion** is the capacity to enter and exit higher states of consciousness (e.g. pure consciousness, cosmic, consciousness, unity, oneness) and other states of trance at one's own discretion (as in deep contemplation, meditation, prayer, etc).

According to Hosseini et al. (2010) spiritual can be viewed as a form of intelligence because it predicts functioning and adaptation and offers capabilities that enable people to solve problems and attain goals.

Recently Kumar and Mehta (2011) have specified spiritual intelligence as the capacity of an individual to possess a socially relevant purpose in life by understanding 'self and having a high degree of conscience, compassion, and commitment to human values. Srivastav & Mishra (2012) have also explored spiritual intelligence as an assistance given to the people in any context (corporate, community or family) to develop their spiritual awareness, capacity and intelligence, and also to use that intelligence to be more effective as an individual, and to expand their capacity to make a great contribution of others.

Spiritual intelligence is effective in people's physical and mental health. Spiritually intelligent individual exhibit mental well-being along with internal and external compassion and reconciliation in any situation (Kates, 2002 & Wigglesworth, 2006). It includes having the feeling of meaning and mission toward life and values, holiness feeling in life, more balanced perception of values and believing to improvement of the world. This intelligence is a set of capabilities and capacities and spiritual resources which lead to adaptability and consequently people mental health (King, 2008; Zohar and Marshall, 2000). Those who possess high spiritual intelligence have the capacity of sublimation and have high tendency towards awareness. They have the capacity to allocate a part of their daily activities to spiritual practice and show virtue like generosity, thanking, humbleness, sympathy and wiseness (Ghobari bonab, 2007).

Therefore, spiritual intelligence represents the ability for integrative perception that see whole beyond its part. This ability assists people on their spiritual path. It may help them perceive the world beyond selfish expectation and corresponding complaints. Spiritual intelligence is the way to assign meaning and feel connected to the power of larger than ourselves.

Resilience

One of the paths through that spiritual intelligence can help to facilitate the psychological well-being lies in increasing the resiliency (Azerbaijani, 2006). The construct of resilience has gained considerable attention over the last four decades since researchers observed that children and youth could cope and adapt in spite of adversity. The term "resilience" is said to have originated from the Latin word "resilire" which means "to recoil or leap back" (Gramezy 1973). It may be thus referred as an individual's tendency to cope with stress and adversity, and this copying may result in the individual "bouncing back" to a previous state of normal functioning, or simply not showing negative effects. Resilience is a broad conceptual umbrella, covering many concepts related to positive patterns of adaptation in the context of adversity. (Masten & Obradovic, 2006).

Empson and Nabuzoka (2004) have referred resilience as "a characteristic of individuals which make them less likely to develop the problem when they have experienced difficult circumstances.". Later, it was recognized that the phenomenon of resilience is relational and therefore must not be conceptualized in term of the trait (Bartlet, 1994). According to Friborg, Hiemdal, Rosenvinge, and Martinussen (2003) resilience process involves the psychological skills and also the possibilities for the individual to take advantage of family, social and external support system in order to cope better with stress.

Resilience is the capacity to cope effectively with the internal stress of their vulnerabilities (such as labile patterns of autonomic reactivity, developmental imbalances, and unusual sensitivities) and external stresses (such as loneliness, major losses, and dissolution of the family). Even though the most stressful experiences in the most terrible homes, some individuals appear to emerge unharmed and to develop a stable, healthy personality (Werner & Smith, 1989).

Resilience could also be explained as the ability to spring back from adversity that interprets the trajectory from risk to problem behaviour or psychopathology and thereby result in adaptive outcomes even in the presence of challenging and threatening circumstances (Zimmerman and Kumar, 1994). It again refers to a class of phenomena characterized by the good outcome in spite of serious threats to adaptation or development (Masten, 2001). It is a dynamic process that can be learned at any given point in life by an individual (Masten, 2001).Thus, resilience can be defined as positive coping with stressful events (Smokowski et al, 1999), or adaptive coping in the face of multiple risk factors. (Waller et al, 2003).

Theoretical Models of Resilience

In past research this area was based on a deficit model, the focus was on problems and psychopathology. Zimmerman and Arunkumar (1994) referred to this as the "pathology of disadvantage" deficit models tend to define individuals in negative terms (Bartely, 2006) and not to expect the individual to succeed. Smith (2006) warns that "we cannot, in good conscience, continue to use a deficit model that has limited value for increasing individuals' resilience to adversity" (p.69). As research continued to evolve, investigator moved away from the pathology-based medical model toward one involving the demonstration of behavioural competence (Kinard, 1998) thus emphasizing the importance of positive adaptation (Cicchetti, 1990; Masten & Braswell, 1991). The strength model, also known as the "asset-based approach" focuses on the strengths and assets of the individual and the resources in his environment that can be mobilized to help him with the problem as opposed to focusing solely on it. By highlighting the universal human capacity for resilience, this model enables ones in preventing, facing, minimizing, overcoming, and even being strengthened or transformed by adversity (Killian, 2004). Richardson (2002) considers this paradigm shift to be a prevalent theme across disciplines.

Besides this important paradigm shift from deficits to strength, another significant advancement from earlier models has been an exploration of the underlying mechanism behind the process of resilience.

Several authors have attempedt to clarify ambiguities related to the concepts. Overviews of these are presented below:

Richardson's (2002) Resiliency Process Model

Richardson (2002) states that when a person experienced difficulty, resiliency becomes a force within him that seeks "self-actualization, altruism, wisdom, and harmony with a spiritual source of strength". He presents resiliency as a simple linear model that depicts a person "passing through the stage of bio psycho- spiritual homeostasis, interactions with life prompts, disruption, and readiness for reintegration and the choice to reintegrate resiliency, back to homeostasis, or with the loss" (p.310). The figure below shows how individuals respond to a disruption in their lives - in enabling, a developmental way of mere survival ways (Boyd & Eckert, 2002).

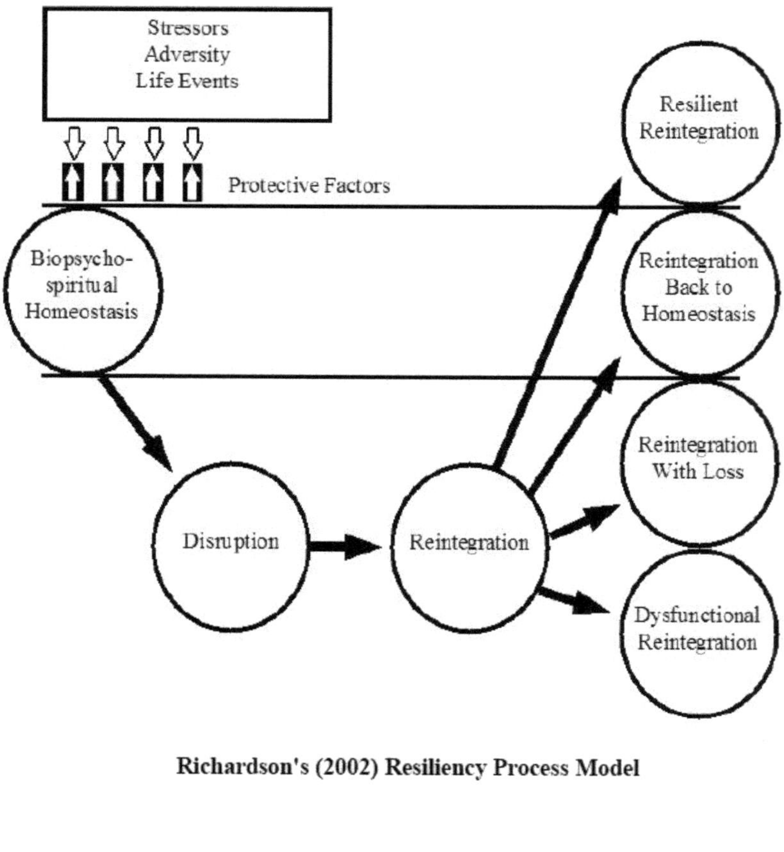

Richardson's (2002) Resiliency Process Model

Richardson (2002), disruptions cause an individual's intact world paradigm to change and this may result in perceived negative and positive outcomes. He cited that being offered a new job, suddenly being countered by a romantic interest, minor accidents or even arguments could be disruptive as they represent change. This model considers resiliency to be a process whereby people have the opportunity to choose consciously or unconsciously the outcomes of disruption. A comfort zone where life seems relatively stable and predictable and healthy development is going on is most preferred (Boyd & Eckart, 2002). Richardson (2002) further points out that people tend to cling to their comfort zones and may turn down opportunities for growth so as to avoid disruptions. He proposes four ways by which individuals counter disruption when it does occur. If people resort to destructive behaviour to deal with the disruption, such as substance use, they are said to be reintegrate dysfunctional. Some fail to recover fully from stressors and lead a life of emptiness and negativism, devoid of motivation, hope or drive, by employing unhealthy coping strategies (Boyd & Eckart, 2002). This is known as reintegration with the loss. The essence of reintegration back to homeostasis is to heal and just get past a disruption. Finally, resilient reintegration is the process by which one experiences growth or insight through disruption (Richardson, 2002). This can be made possible through learning, and by gaining deeper insights into the situation that makes one stronger, more knowing, loving and resilient (Boyd & Eckart, 2002). This also explains why some people become stronger after experiencing greatly challenging disruption and have a potential for change at one point in time in an individual's life, there may be multiple disruptive and re integrative ongoing growth opportunities that may be happening simultaneously.

Rew and Horner's (2003) Youth Resilience Framework

This model addresses individuals socio cultural risk and protective factors that can promote or hinder positive and negative health outcomes in adolescence. Assuming that risk and protective factors are present throughout an individual's life. Rew and Horner (2003) state that resilience may be considered as the outcome of triadic influence of risk, protection, and interventions.

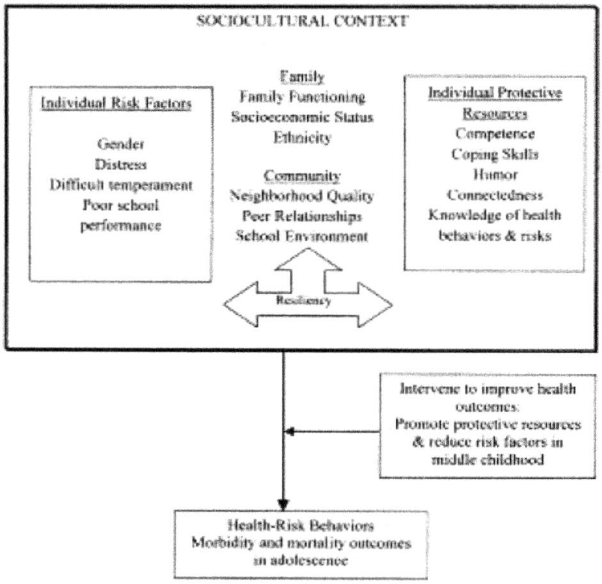

Rew and Horner's (2003) Youth Resilience Framework

Rew and Horner (2003) pointed out that those with many risk factor and few protective resources are vulnerable to adverse health outcomes in adolescence. Factors such as increased distress and poor school performance are associated with multiple health-risk behaviours, including tobacco and alcohol use, weapon-carrying, or suicide attempts (Rew & Horner, 2003). The author suggests that early intervention enhances protective resources, in spite of multiple individuals and socio cultural risk factors, must be developed to promote the health and well-being of adolescents.

Kumpfer's (1999) Framework of Resilience

Kumpfer (1999) proposed that when individuals encounter stressful situations, they experience a person-environment transactional process which is influenced by environmental contexts and personal resiliency factors. This model is an initiating event or a stressor that signifies disruption in the individual's homeostatic environment but at the same time, also sets in motion the process of re-establishing the disrupted life of the individual. This process ends in an outcome that may be resilient reintegration or maladaptive reintegration, the latter implying non-resilience.

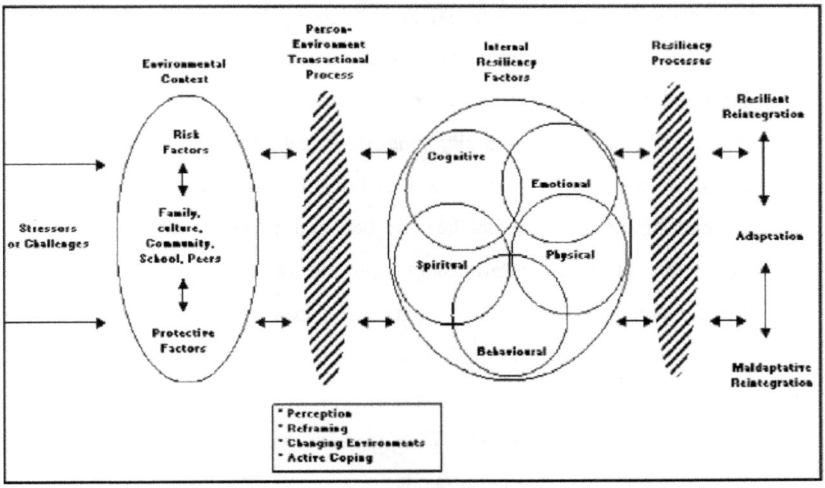

Kumfer's (1999) Framework of Resilience

The major predictors of resilience according to this model are stressors or challenges, environmental context, person-environmental context, person-environment transaction process, internal resilience factor and outcomes of the interactions, resilience process, and adaptive, resilient reintegration or maladaptive non-resilient reintegration (Mampane 2005). Major factors in the person-environment transactional process include perception, reframing, changing the environment, and active coping. Perception refers to the way that people view the stressful situation. Reframing is the individual's tendency to change the meaning of the situation. Changing environments refers to people's efforts to bring about a change in the environment. Active coping refers to strategies that are characterized by problem-solving, seeking social support, and drawing meaning out of experience (Li, 2008).

Personality

Personality is mainly connected with social and psychological aspects, like sense of dignity, self-appraisal, value orientations, beliefs, the principles by which the person lives moral, aesthetic, socio-political and different social positions, convictions and ideals, and additionally the character, the special features of intellect, the style and independence of thinking, the specific nature of emotional make-up, willpower, cast of mind and feelings, social position. Personality involves collective principles that merge biological and social in a single whole and also all the psychological processes, qualities, and states that regulate behaviour, giving it a certain consistency and stability in relation to the rest of the world, to other people and itself. Personality is a socially historical, naturally conditioned and individuality expressed being. The core of personality is not its physical nature but its socio-psychological properties and the mechanism of its mental life and behaviour. The personality is an individual's expression of social relationships and functions, a subject of cognition and transformation of the world of rights and duties of ethical, aesthetic and all other social standards. When we think about personality, we have in mind its social, moral, psychological and aesthetic qualities crystallized in a human being's intellectual world. Personality is made up of the characteristic patterns of thought, feelings, and behaviour that make a person unique. In addition, personality arises from within the individual and remains fairly consistent throughout life. Some main characteristics of personality include consistency, psychological, and physiological developments reflected through behaviour and action and finally the multiple expressions.

Thus the term personality was understood by different psychologists. Personality is the dynamic organization within the individual of those psychophysical systems that determine his unique adjustments to his environment Gordon W. Allport (1961).

Personality is a stable set of characteristics and tendencies that determine those commonalities and differences in the psychological behavior (thoughts, feelings, and actions) of people that have continuity in time and that may not be easily understood as the sole result of the social and biological pressures of the moment Salvatore Maddi (1998). Personality is the dynamic organization within the individual of that psychophysical system that determines his unique adjustments to the environment and his characteristic behaviour of thought (Allport1937, 1961).

Personality is an important determining factor for well-being (Gilovich & Eibach, 2001). It refers to an individual's characteristic patterns of thought, emotion and behaviour together with psychological mechanism i.e. hidden or not behind those patterns (Funder, 2004).

Larsen and Buss (2005) specified "personality as the set of psychological traits and mechanism within the individual that are organized and relatively enduring that influences his or her interaction with, and adoptions too, the intra-psychic, physical and social environments".

Mayer (2007) defined that personality is the organized developing system within the individual that represents the collective action of individual's major psychological subsystems.

Costa & McCrae (1992) have described personality on the basis of five domains i.e. extroversion, neuroticism (or emotional instability), agreeableness, openness, and conscientiousness known as the "Big Five" theory of personality (Costa &McCrae, 1992; John, 1990). These Five domains are as follows:

(i) **Neuroticism**: It is the general tendency to experience negative effects such as fear, sadness, embarrassment, anger, guilt, and disgust is the core of the Neuroticism domain. However, neuroticism includes more than susceptibility to psychological distress because disruptive emotion interferes with adaptation. The people high on neuroticism are also prone to have irrational ideas, cannot control their impulses, and to cope more poorly than other stress.

(ii) **Extroversion-** Extraverts are, sociable, but sociability is only one of the traits that comprise the domain of extraversion. In addition to liking people and preferring large group and gatherings, extroverts are also assertive, active and talkative. They like excitement and stimulation and tend to be cheerful in disposition. They are upbeat, energetic, and optimist.

(iii) **Openness**: It is the third major dimension of personality. The component of openness is dynamic imagination, aesthetic sensitivity, attentiveness to inner feelings, and preference for variety, intellectual curiosity, and independence of judgment. Open individuals are curious about both inner and outer world, and their lives are experimentally richer. They are willing to entertain newest concepts and unconventional values, and that they experience both positive and negative emotions more keenly than to close individuals.

(iv) **Agreeableness**: It is primarily a dimension of interpersonal tendencies. The agreeable person is fundamentally altruistic. This type of person is sympathetic to other and eager to help them and believes that other will be equally helpful in return. These domains describe personality as both socially preferable and psychologically healthier.

(v) **Conscientiousness:** Self-control is the basic tendency of Conscientiousness. Self-control refers to an active process of planning, organizing and carrying out the task and individual differences in this tendency are the basis of Conscientiousness. The Conscientious individual is purposeful strong-willed and determined.

Mental Health

Psychological well- being may be defined as the subjective feeling of contentment, happiness, satisfaction to life experience and of one's role in the world of work, sense of achievement, utility, belongingness, and no distress, dissatisfaction, worry etc. Mental health is a broad concept and has been one of the major subject of psychological interest and recently also been one of the major subject of psychological interest and academic interest. World Health Organization (WHO, 2001) defined "Mental Health as a state of complete physical, mental and social well-being and not merely the absence of disease or infirmity". This definition elaborates that mental health can be conceptualized as a state of well-being in which the individual realizes his or her own abilities, can cope with the normal stresses of life, can work productively and fruitfully and is able to make to contribute to his or her community. It has always been easier to define mental health through mental illness; however, it has now been recognized that mental health is more than the absence of mental illness. Good Mental health involves positive psychosocial skills; qualities that are present in resilient people as well (Beardslee, 1989). Mental health involves not only freedom from mental disorders, such as depression, anxiety, psychotic condition, or personality problems, but also the regular experience of positive emotions, such as joy, wonder, happiness, satisfaction, meaning, purpose and hope. Mental health is important as it affects everything one does i.e., how one sleeps, what one eats, the risk one will take and the type of thing one does to relax and enjoy one.

Mental health approach in education has emerged as a strongest movement that has spread to all enlightened system of the world.

The definition of positive mental health from Mental Health Foundation (2002) encompasses aspects of both emotional well-being and social functioning. This includes self-confidence, assertiveness, empathy, the capacity to develop emotionally, creatively, intellectually, and spiritually, the capacity to initiate and sustain mutually satisfying personal relationships, and capacity to face problems, resolve and learn from them, to use and enjoy solitude, to play and have fun, to laugh at oneself and at the world.

In general terms, mental health is full and harmonious functioning of whole personality. Meninger (1945) defines mental health as the adjustment of human beings to the world and to each other with a maximum of effectiveness and happiness. It is the ability to maintain an even temper, an alert intelligence, socially considerate behaviour and a happy dispositionl. Jahoda (1958), an advocate of the concept of positive mental health said that it means a successful synthesis of the factors, which the people are, where he is and what he wishes to be. The behaviour of a person is determined by concepts unifying look on, life, possessions of a long range of goals, and appropriate connections with the past are the characteristics of a healthy person.

Jahoda (1958) has conceptualized following six aspects of positive mental health:

- **Attitudes of an individual towards his own self**: the accessibility of the self to consciousness, the correctness of the self-concept, and its relation to the sense of identity and the acceptance by the individual of his own self.
- **Growth, development, or self-actualization**: the extent to which the individual utilizes his abilities.
- **Integration**: the extent to which the psychic forces are balanced.
- **Autonomous**: is self-reliant and is able to decide what suits his own needs best.
- **Perception of reality**: is the freedom from need distortion and existence of empathy.

- **Environmental mastery:** is an adequacy in interpersonal relationships adaptation and adjustment and efficiency in problem-solving.

Looking after one's mind is equally important as looking after one's body. As part of one's overall health, mental and emotional health is a necessary condition to enable one's life successfully. Mental health is the emotional and spiritual resilience that allows to enjoy life and to survive pain, suffering, and disappointment. It is a positive sense of well-being and an underlying belief in one's own and others dignity and worth. Mental health is about

- how one feels inside
- balancing one's emotions and having control on them
- self-esteem and confidence
- being comfortable with whom they are
- coping with one's feelings and building up resilience on one's "bounce-back ability"

Maslow and Mittelmann (1951) have suggested the following criteria for normal psychological health:

- the adequate feeling of security.
- adequate self-evaluation.
- adequate spontaneity and emotionality.
- efficient conduct with reality.
- adequate bodily desire and the ability to gratify them.
- adequate self-knowledge.
- integration and consistency of personality.
- adequate life goals.
- ability to learn from experience.
- ability to satisfy the requirements of the group.
- adequate emancipation from the group or culture.

Allport has given (1961) six silent features for a sound healthy personality:

- Extension of the sense of self.
- Capable of intimacy, respect, and compassion when relating to others.
- Emotional security (self-acceptance).
- Realistic perception and skills.
- Self-objectification, i.e. insight and humor.
- A unifying philosophy of a life a sense of direction and purpose in life.

Korchin (1976) had given the idea that psychological health should focus on the ideal state, i.e. his emphasis was on the "positive well-being" rather than on disease, statistical or conformity criteria. Mental health must be defined as a state of physical, social and psychological well-being rather than simply as an absence of illness or sickness. He also stressed the importance of the development of human potentials illness which is considered to be a reflection of individual response to stress and change in the social cultural, economic and psychological atmosphere. Adolescents account for about 1/5th of India's population. In recent times, newspapers reported at least cases of suicides and attempts which mainly circumvented school life. This is particularly true of class X and intermediate or pre university (PUC) students, who get frustrated because of the pressure imposed by the teachers and parents and factors like competition high ambitions etc. Thus are more prone to a vulnerability which may lead to ill health, negative feeling or suicides.

At least one in five children and adolescents may express mental health problems in a year and in the United States, it is estimated that one in ten children and adolescents suffer from mental illness severe enough to cause some level of impairment. It is estimated that six to nine million children and adolescents in the United States have mental or behavioural problems. Indian Council of Medical Research reported that about 12.8 per cent of children (1-16 years) suffer from mental health problems in India.

According to Dandapani, (2000) mental health refers to full and harmonious functioning of our total personality as well as to our bio-socio-psychological and spiritual well-being. It is associated with the prevention of mental disorders, also the treatment and rehabilitation of individuals affected by mental disorders. Mental health is a term used to describe how well the individual is adjusted to the demands and opportunities of life.

The World Health Organization (The World Health Report, 2001) defined mental health as "a state of well-being in which the individual realizes his or her own abilities, can cope with the normal stresses of life, can work productively and fruitfully, and is able to make a contribution to his or her community".

Coleman (1970) defined mental health as "the ability to balance feelings, desires ambitions and ideas in one's daily livings and to face and accept the realities of life. It is the habit of work and attitude towards people and things that bring maximum satisfaction and happiness to the individuals". In the book entitled 'Mental Hygiene in Public Health", Lewkan (2006) has written that a mentally healthy individual is one who himself is satisfied, lives peacefully with his neighbors, makes healthy citizens of his children and even after performing these fundamental duties has enough energy left to do something for the benefit of society. Emotional mental disorders are the leading cause of disabilities worldwide. Investigating the degree and severity of untreated emotional mental disorders throughout the world is a top priority of the World Mental Health (WMH) survey initiative, which was created in 1998 by the World Health Organization (WHO) (Thornicroft, 2007).

CHAPTER- II

REVIEW OF LITERATURE

An exhaustive survey of the related studies was conducted, after having selecting the topic an intensive review of survey literature was completed. Available journals, periodicals, periodicals, reference materials, encyclopedias and book from different sources have been consulted for this purpose. A systematic reporting of this review is being presented in the following section. As the research studies related to the variables of present study have gone on since long, consequently the corpus of researches in India and aboard. Therefore it was not possible to report all the studies. A systematic reporting of this review is being presented in the following section.

Studies Related to Spiritual Intelligence and Mental Health

In a study Lotfi and Sayyar (2008) have evaluated the correlation between spiritual intelligence and mental health of middle adolescents and they established the notion that there is a considerable relationship between spiritual intelligence and mental health. In an additional study, Steward and Joe (2006) have also set up that spiritual sense is remarkably correlated to mental health and compatibility and religious students are more attuned than rest and enjoyed from the highest educational result.

Larson, Sherrill, Lyons, Craigie, Thielman, Greenwold, et al. (1992) studied a 12-year follow up of all articles appearing in American Journal of Psychiatry and Archives of General Psychiatry and discovered that 72% of the spiritual obligation variables were advantageous to mental health; input in religious services, social hold up, prayer and rapport with God were favorable in 92% of citations.

In an assessment, Elmer, Mac Donald, and Friedman (2003) exposed that spirituality has an optimistic authority on physical condition. It plays a function in declining disease rate and longer existence. Those human being who were internally slanting appear to exceptionally take actions about interference, optimistically covenant with disturbance (Emmons, 2000) and have reduced rate of depression (MacDonald & Friedman, 2002). Desrosiers and Miller (2007) examined 615 young girls, in which they showed that with stronger religious constituent (faith) they behave more authoritative in dealing with personal and educational stresses, also they are less horizontal to syndrome and they have higher psychosomatic well-being.

In another study Lazar (2009) examined the association flanked by multidimensional measure of spiritual orientation and measures of psychological functioning amongst a sample of secular Israeli Jews, One hundred and twelve research participants responded to the Spiritual Orientation Inventory (Elkins et. al., 1988) to self report measures of dejection and life contentment. Noteworthy associations stuck between total spirituality and both despair and life satisfactions were enclosed even after controlling for religiousness. Partial correlations exposed that life coherency, intrinsic values, and experimental aspects of spirituality were interrelated to these procedures even after calculating for other dimensions of spirituality. Deterioration analysis established the unique endowment of these three aspects of spirituality to the forecast of despair and of inherent spiritual ideas to the prediction of life contentment.

Hassan (2009) in his study indicated that students with elevated levels of SQ are found to be extra convinced in taking an action and more responsive towards their environment. Consequently, they are capable to locate themselves within any circumstance and fabricate a sooth stipulation that increases their accomplishment in education. Spiritual intelligence helps a person age to walk around his self-potential. Researches in the mental condition bring to a close that those who are fewer spiritual may practice more depression and emerge to recuperate from depression more leisurely (Braam, et al., 1997; Braam et al., 2001).

Spiritual intelligence is one of the respective types of intelligence that can be developed independently and bring to psychological well-being and overall healthy human development (Perez, 2012). Previous findings on the association between spirituality and mental health have found that people who consider themselves as spiritually experienced potentially benefitted in terms of low rates of psychological distress, more satisfaction with life and more likely to be high achievers of their goals compared to others who are not spiritual (Corrigan et al., 2003). The role played by spirituality in promoting mental health among different sections of the populations is being widely researched and the findings are impressive with regards to positive associations between the two (Corrigan et al., 2003). Nelms (2005) also conducted a study on the relationship between spirituality and the health of college student in a university setting and found that the relationship between the self-reported level of spirituality and the health status of college is positive relationship between spirituality and mental health. A review by Mishra and Vashist (2014) also revealed that spiritual intelligence has a significant influence on the quality of life and success for adolescents in the 21st century which needs to be understood. Spiritual functions including spiritual intelligence and its components can be used as a possible instrument to increase individual's mental health (West, 2004).

In another review article about adolescence, Hosseini et al. (2010) have explained its relation to spiritual intelligence and the related theories. Spiritual intelligence had a significant influence on the quality of life and it goes without saying that adolescence is a sensitive period which requires specific training to make a brighter future and be exposed to the difficulties. Spirituality can be viewed as a form of intelligence because it predicts functioning and adaptation and offers capabilities that enable people to solve problems and attain goals. The results showed that conceiving spirituality as a sort of intelligence extended the psychologist's conception of spirituality and allowed its association with the rational cognitive processes like goal achievement and problem-solving. It was also concluded that emotional intelligence allows a person to judge in which situation he was involved and then to behave appropriately within it while spiritual intelligence allows a person us to ask if he wants to be in this particular situation in the first place.

Kezdy, Martos, and Boland (2011) investigated and evaluated the relationship between spiritual attitudes and mental health in the adolescents as optimistic and noteworthy. Koenig (2012) conducted a cross-cultural study by which he presented that western and eastern spirituality in all cultures has positive consequence in growing modification and comfort. Susana, Ramirez, Macedo, and Sales (2012) carried out a longitudinal learning by which he showed that spirituality based coping is allied with the amplified quality of life and well-being in patients with renal ailment and dialysis. In a study Yahaya, Momtaz, Othman, Sulaiman & Arisah (2012) examined the impact of spirituality on adolescents' mental health problems and they found that existential well-being and religious well-being were statistically related with lower odds of mental health problems. Thus, spirituality as a confidence factor might help children to cope with physical and psychological changes through adolescence, fruitfully. Recently Babanazari et al. (2012) analyzed the association between spiritual intelligence and contentment for adolescents on a sample of 221 high school students. The outcome of the reading exposed that there was a positive relationship between spiritual intelligence and contentment. Regression investigation showed that consciousness sensing, mystery sensing, value sensing and community sensing considerably projected gladness.

Shabani et al. (2011) in a srudy exemplified whether spiritual intelligence and emotional intelligence can be measured as a predictor for mental health. Also, this study explored the moderating possessions of gender on the link between spiritual intelligence and emotional intelligence with mental health among high school students. The participants were 247 high school students, (124 male and 123 female, 14-17 years old). The study intends an exposit facto and tested the substitute hypotheses. Three applicable and consistent instruments were used for evaluation, viz., spiritual intelligence emotional intelligence and mental health. The results established that mental health can be controlled by spiritual intelligence and emotional intelligence. In accumulation, the moderating consequence of gender on the rapport of spiritual intelligence and emotional intelligence with mental health was not recognized.

An investigation outcome by Pargament and Smith in 1998 demonstrated the positive possessions of spirituality on individual's adjustment and coping with social anxiety and life stressors. Studies have also set up correlations between spirituality and mental health variables such as stress (Woodbury, 1992); anxiety (Alvordo, 1995), emotional instability and mood disorders (Jang & Johnson, 2004; Leach & Lark, 2004), depression (Genia, 2001; & Koenig, 2007), neuroticism & substance abuse (Elmer, MacDonald, & Friedman, 2003).

Singh and Singh (2011) had an intention to observe the mental health of senior secondary school students in relation to spiritual interference, gender, and religion. The study sample comprised of 934 adolescent students from different schools affiliated to Punjab School Education Board. The result showed that mental health of senior secondary school students with high and average spiritual intelligence was better than senior secondary school students with low spiritual intelligence.

Pant and Srivastava (2014) also conducted a study on college students and reported that spiritual intelligence and mental health are correlated significantly, and there is a significant relationship between spiritual intelligence and quality of life and finally, mental health and quality of life are correlated significantly with each other among college students. Spiritual intelligence and mental health are positively correlated among adolescents (Singh, 2014).

In others populations it was also revealed a significant positive correlation between spiritual and nurse's public health (Akbarizadeh, Bagheri, Hatami, & Hajiwandy, 2011). Jain & Purohit (2006) studied the spiritual intelligence of elderly people for this purpose. 200 senior citizens were selected from different living status i.e. living with family and living in old age homes. Findings suggested that no significant difference was found between senior citizens living with family & living in old age homes regarding overall spiritual-intelligence. On the other hand findings showed significant differences at many domains of spiritual intelligence such as, GOD and religiosity, soul, self-awareness, interpersonal relations, spirituality in leadership, helping behaviour, flexibility, ability to use and overcome suffering, ability to transcend pain and being spiritually intelligent about death.

Nasruddin, Husain, and Hameed (2011) measured the level of spiritual intelligence among male and female students studying in professional and non-professional courses at the University of Malaya. The main effects of gender and vocational stream and their interaction effects were not found to be significant. Some findings revealed that professional and non-professional students significantly differed with respect to spiritual intelligence. More specifically, professional students were found to have higher spiritual intelligence than non-professional students. When the investigators compared on four factors of spiritual intelligencei.e., critical existential thinking (CET), personal meaning production (PMP), transcendental awareness (TA) and conscious state expansion (CSE) resulted again that two groups differed significantly on these factors (Hilal & Siddiqui, 2013). Ahmadi and Kajbaf (2008) found that there is no difference in different educational groups in terms of spiritual intelligence but in an extensive analysis of spiritual intelligence.

In another study Hariri and Zarrin- Abadi (2011) demonstrated that there is a meaningful relationship between educational field and spiritual intelligence. In a recent study, Anjumn (2015) compared professional and non-professional course students on measures of spiritual intelligence, academic stress, life satisfaction and mental health. It was found that the professional courses students showed relatively low level of spiritual intelligence, academic stress, and better mental health. In contrast to it, the non-professional courses students showed a higher level of spiritual intelligence, academic stress, and poor mental health. So far as their life satisfaction was concerned they did not differ significantly but on other measures both the groups differed significantly.

The review of the literature shows that there is a positive relationship between spiritual intelligence and mental health of adolescents. One of the reasons may be that spiritual intelligence as a psychological benefit to an individual provides people a sense of purpose and meaning in life and spiritual values honesty, patience, kindness, joy, hope, love, etc may help the person to cope with the different and stressful situation. Spiritual intelligence helps people to reduce their negative emotions and benefit from appropriate strategies to manage stress and solve life problems and to minimize anxiety. When spiritual intelligence is high, we appear to be intellectual and have proper behaviour and better mental health of individuals. However, when spiritual intelligence is low, people appear to have problematic behaviour. An individual with high spiritual intelligence demonstrates higher measures of satisfaction and performance. Thus spiritual intelligence could be helpful in conflict management and peaceful co-existence in the society as it is a personal quality which enables the person to maintain both inner and outer peace and display love regardless of the circumstances whether stress or acute conflict.

Studies Related to Gender Differences in Spiritual Intelligence

A good number of studies have been conducted in India in relation to spiritual intelligence and mental health and it shows positive relationship. Gupta (2012) investigated a study on the relationship between spiritual intelligence and emotional intelligence with self efficacy and self regulation among college students. The findings revealed that spiritual intelligence and emotional intelligence were positively and significantly correlated with self efficacy and self regulation. The significant difference was found between male and female students regarding emotional intelligence, self efficacy and self regulation. It was also found that male students were better in spiritual intelligence and emotional intelligence as compared to female students.

Study conducted by Jeloudar et.al. (2010) and Kushwaha (2012) on B.Ed students (150 male and 150 female) reported that female has a higher level of spiritual intelligence as compared to male. Similarly, Singh (2011) found that girls had significantly higher level of spiritual intelligence and altruism as compared to boys. A study made by Khan and Singh (2013) indicates that significant gender differences were found among male and female teachers on spirituality and females were found higher on spirituality than males. A recent study by Nangia and Kushwaha (2014) was conducted on the spiritual intelligence of school students. The results revealed that female students have higher spiritual intelligence as compared to male students. Further, the results revealed that students studying in government schools were found to be more in spiritual intelligence than students studying in private schools.

However, in another study done by Siddiqui (2013) to see the effect of achievement motivation and gender on spiritual intelligence reported no gender effect on spiritual intelligence. A study also done by Kaur and Singh (2013) revealed that there is no significant effect of gender, locality and family status on the factors underlying spiritual intelligence except in the domain of extrasensory perception (males were greater than females) and mindfulness (high class showed higher than middle class) in case of engineering students and community (middle class was greater than high class), trauma (middle class show higher than high class) and intellectuality (middle class was greater than high class) in case of teacher training students.

Similarly, Nazam (2014) conducted a study on graduate students (19 to 24 years) to see the gender difference on spiritual intelligence between adolescents. The findings of the research were as follows i.e., the important distinction was found among the two groups, on subscales, namely, personal meaning production (PMP), conscious state expansion (CSE), transcendental awareness (TA) and critical existential thinking (CET) and composite scores on spiritual intelligence. In the same manner Jafari et al (2014) also reported that no significant differences were found between female and male students on the scores of spiritual intelligence. It was again justified by study of Kotnala, (2015) finding out the spiritual intelligence among graduate students. The findings of the study revealed that there is no significant difference between male and female students on conscious state expansion, critical existential thinking, personal meaning production and transcendental awareness of spiritual intelligence. Whereas, Bhagwan (2015) did a comparative study on male and female graduate colleges on spiritual intelligence. Finding show the significant gender difference in spiritual intelligence.

The review related to gender signifies that there is significant difference between male and female adolescents on spiritual intelligence. It is also found that spirituality influences the psychological health and physical health of individuals since many decades.

Studies Related to Resilience and Mental Health

Many studies have reported that resilient individuals possess better mental health than others. Fergusson and Horwood (2003) in studying childhood adversity found that resilience was related to absence of symptomatology such as depression, anxiety, conduct disorders, alcohol and drug dependence, suicidal behaviour and criminal offending. According to Stewart, Reid, and Mangham (1998), health can embrace the feelings of connectedness, control, meaning and self-efficacy which all are relevant factors in resilience. They cited that the relationship of resilience and health is elucidated in discussions of risk factors, protective factors and resilient outcomes in resiliency literature.

In a study, it was found that the individuals who got highest scores in resilience have lowest levels of depression, anxiety and obsession symptoms (Hjemdal, Vogel, Solem, Hagen and Stiles, 2011). In the same way, resilience is among the factors which help to confront and adapting to difficult and tension-making situations of life and protects people against pathological disorders and life difficulties (Rutter M. 1985). Baldwin et al., (1993) have reported that non-resilient children have lower mental health scores than resilient children.

Roy, Sarchiapone, and Carli (2007) administered the Connor-Davidson Resilience Scale on 100 abstinent substance dependent outpatients and found that those who had suicidal ideation were scored significantly low on resilience than that patients who had never attempted suicide. This suggests the possibility that low resilience may be related to poor mental health (depression and suicidal ideation in this case). Vaishnavi, Connor, and Davidson (2007) in their study agreed that increased resilience may be related to neuropsychiatric disease prevention after exposure to environmental stressors.

Some researchers have contended that adolescents described as resilient on one dimension may still be vulnerable on another. The latter being the area of mental health. In an investigation on emotional distress among inner-city adolescents thought to be resilient, the children exhibited both high levels of stress and high levels of social competence (Luthar, 1991). Interestingly, resilient youths were found to be more depressed than those who were highly competent but from low-stress backgrounds. In addition, both groups had comparable levels of internalizing symptoms, such as anxiety and depression. Similar findings were reported by Luthar, Doernberger, and Zigler (1993) who observed that 85% of the inner-city children who seemed resilient based on one domain of social competency, showed significant signs of impairment on one or more domains six months later. This led the investigators to conclude that "resilience is not a uni dimensional construct" (Luthar, Doernberger & Zigler, 1993). Zucker, Wong, Puttler, and Fitzgerald (2003) found that preschoolers who did not show obvious signs of disturbance were found to experience internalizing symptoms. Later, Luthar (2006) cited that high empathic self-efficacy among adolescents was related to high prosocial behaviour and less delinquency among both males and females. These findings suggest that even though some high-risk students can seem to be resilient in terms of their behaviour, whilst meeting societal expectations or showing competence, many of these students might still struggle with inner distress in the form of problems such as depression and anxiety (Luthar, 2006). Luthar and Cicchetti (2000) again added that internalizing symptoms if left unattended can eventually derail apparently in resilient trajectories. This is yet another example of the controversy that attends the concept of resiliency (Lazarus, 2004). In other words, poor mental health may be the price one pays for being resilient.

In a study Hartly (2011) examined the relationship between measures of interpersonal resilience, intrapersonal resilience, and mental health and it was examined with respect to academic and social integration. Resilience was defined as "the process of, capacity for, or outcome of successful adaptation despite challenging or threatening circumstances." It was found that there was a strong statistical correlation between the inter-and-intrapersonal (tendency, tolerance of stress and spirituality) resilience factors and mental health. Besharat (2008) demonstrated an inverse correlation between resilience and distress, depression, anxiety and general health problems and reported that resilience was positively associated with psychological well-being and negatively associated with psychological distress, depression, and anxiety. Psychological health and vulnerability indices are influenced by different levels of resilience through self-esteem, personal competence and tenacity, tolerance of negative affect, control, and spirituality. Hamid, Keikhosravani, Babamiri, and Dehghani (2012) investigated the relationship between mental health, spiritual intelligence, and resiliency among the Kermanshah Medical Science University. The results indicated that there was a positive significant relationship between mental health and resiliency.

In an interesting observation by Hunter and Chandler (1999), $10^{th}$and 11^{th}grade volunteers from an inner-city, vocational high-school in New England were observed Wagnuild and Young's resiliency Scale (1993) was administered to measure their perception of resilience. Focus groups, structured and unstructured interviews and written stories were used to gather phenomenological data. Despite the stressful world in which the participants lived, the adolescents marked themselves as "resilient". However, they believed that being resilient was to be disconnected from others because they could not trust, isolated because they had no support systems and insulated because the emotional pain was too much to bear.

According to Hudson (2007), mental health professionals must focus on what makes a difference in the lives of resilient children and adolescents. In this context, Luthar and Cicchetti (2000) pointed out that most of the existing resiliency programs attempted to foster academic or job skills or reduce behaviours that are disruptive to others (conduct or antisocial problems). However, there is little cognizance of the reality "that a child's emotional state also affects his or her ability to achieve the level of social and cognitive competence to learn" (Knitzer, 2000).

Researches have shown strong linkages between resilience and mental health and there are positive linkages between resilience and mental health. Literature also reveals that resilient individuals possess better mental health than others.

Druss and Douglas (1988) studied the nature and source of resilience in three individuals facing serious illness and disability. They focused on the relationship between "healthy denial" and adaptive responses to illness. These three live accounts described how the individuals remained optimistic in the face of adversity as they continued to engage in productive activities. They denied the most threatening implications and emotional impact of their condition. They referred to their illness not as a "narcissistic injury but as an opportunity for personal growth". Moreover, these three individuals felt no self-pity, anger, or envy towards those who were healthy. They were found to exhibit the resilient attributes of equanimity, perseverance, self-reliance, meaningfulness and existential (Wagnild & Young, 1993).

Fredrickson, Tugade, Waugh, and Larkin (2003) attempted to find out if positive emotions buffer resilient people from depression and help them thrive in those circumstances. In order to examine this hypothesis, pre and post-crisis tests were conducted on 18 and 28 women. Although positive emotions are often considered to be subtle and fleeting experiences, making it difficult to envision them as having much importance in the face of sudden trauma, the results of the study illustrate that positive emotions hold depressive symptoms. Similarly in another experiment, Tugade and Fredrickson (2004) used a multi-method approach to predict that resilient people use positive emotions and find positive meaning in stressful encounters. By examining psychological resilience from subjective, cognitive and physiological angles, the investigators discovered that resilient individual experience of positive emotions enabled them to pursue novel and creative thoughts and actions during times of stress. It was thus concluded that with time, they may be able to build an ability of effective coping resources through exploration and experimentation that help buffer against negative emotional life experiences both psychologically and physiologically.

In recent years, the association between resilience and mental health has been studied extensively. In a recent study Khordzanganeh, F., Heidarie, A. R., and Naderi, F. (2014) explored the relationship between emotional intelligence, happiness and resiliency with mental health in male and female high school students of Ramhormoz city. Sample of 365 students (223 girls and 142 boys) were selected by multistage cluster sampling method. The results showed that the correlation between emotional intelligence, happiness, and resiliency with mental health are significant. Also among the predictor variables, resiliency has the stronger ability to predict mental health than happiness and emotional intelligence.

In an another recent study by Mc Gilivray and Pidgeon (2015) on Australian University students investigated the attributes of resilient university students, by comparing the differences between high and low resilient students on levels of reported psychological distress, sleep disturbances and mindfulness. A total of 89 university students participated in the study aged between 18 to 57 years. Results showed that university students with high levels of resilience reported significantly lower levels of psychological distress and significantly higher levels of mindfulness, compared to university students reporting low levels of resilience. The findings also add to the extent the knowledge of resilience and provide support for universities to develop strategies that promote resilience in university students to reduce the risk of students developing mental health problems, thus enabling students to flourish under academic pressures. In a study Kirmani, Sharma, Anas, and Sanam (2015) examined the hope, resilience and subjective well-being in a group of college-going adolescent girls. A sample of 98 college-going adolescent girls from one of the government universities at Aligarh city was selected using convenience sampling technique. The findings indicate significant positive relationships among hope and resilience, hope and subjective well-being and resilience and subjective well-being.

In a very recent study by Hajizadeh, Khalili, Haghighi, &Malekpour, (2016) revealed the role of resiliency and quality of life on the mental health of third-grade high school students in Shiraz. For this purpose, among third-year high school students of Shiraz, 340 students (178 females and 162 males) were selected. The results showed that resiliency variable has a positive and significant relationship with all components of quality of life (physical health, psychological health, social relationships, and environment). There is a significant relationship between the components of mental health (stress, anxiety, depression) with resiliency, quality of life and its components. Also resilience and quality of life were emerged as the significant predictors for all the components of mental health i.e., depression, stress, anxiety. Similar in a study, Bastaminia, A., Hashemi, F. B., Alizadeh, M., and Dastoorpoor, M. (2016) observed the significant inverse correlation between resilience and all subscales of general health.

Thus, it can be observed that the majority of studies show that resilience is directly related to mental health. Resilience could also be explained as the ability to spring back from adversity that interprets the trajectory from risk to problem behaviour or psychopathology and thereby result in adaptive outcomes even in the presence of challenging and threatening circumstances (Zimmerman and Arun Kumar, 1994).

It may be thus deduced from literature presented above that resilience is an important part of life and resilient individuals are expected to show better mental health and competence as compared to those who are low on resilience. People with higher resiliency represent higher degree of mental health and also resiliency can strengthen people in the face of mental stresses, tension and depression.

Studies Related to Gender Differences in Resilience

Resilience promotion (Holmes & Jones, 2009) upholds that building resilience needs to be gender-sensitive. Researches in resiliency demonstrated obligating evidence that many factors may help students at the risk of failure to exposes competence (Garmenzy, Masten, & Tellegen, 1984; Rutter, 1979). In resilience, gender has been found to be one such determinant (Grotberg, 1997; Masten et al., 1988). In their analysis of gender variations of resiliency Werner and Smith (1992) discovered that not only were males and females likely to differ in the ages at which they were most susceptible to stress, but they also were likely to differ in the ways in which they coped with it. Most of the longitudinal studies have found females to show more resilience as compared to males (Rutter, 1985; Werner & Smith, 1982). McGloin and Widom (2001) in their attempt to measure resilience in terms of successful functioning found that females were likely to meet the criterion for overall resilience (success in six out of eight domains) than males and those females were successful across a greater number all of domains than males. .

Empirical literature also indicates that females have higher resilience than males in diverse groups such as children (Werner, 1985; Sun and Stewart, 2007; Riches et al., 2009), adolescents (Chung and Elias, 1996; Hair et al., 2001; Hampel and Petermann, 2005; Arokiaraj et al., 2011) and adults (Netuveli et al., 2008; Wagnield, 2011; Ma et al., 2013).

Based on above data there were studies by Somchit and Sriyaporn's(2004) on 9-16-year-olds children, Banyard and Cantor's (2004) investigation on college students, and Sun and Stewart's (2007) on 8-12-year-olds. Findings of all studies reported that females showed greater resilience than males among all group. Kaur and Kaur (2012) also reported that female adolescents found to be more resilient than male adolescents.

Studies have also explored the contradictory finding to explain resilience. In a study Morales' (2008) on American and Hispanic participants revealed that females faced greater resistance than males in the pursuit of their career goals also. Grotberg (1997) agrees that despite perceiving more adversity than males, females were found to use resilience factors such as trusting relationships and finding support more than males. On the other hand, study by Al-Naser and Sandman (2000) also investigated to identify resilience characteristics in college students of Kuwait University, following the Iraqi invasion of Kuwait in 1990. Sample consists of 495 male and female students. Result found that males have scored higher on resilience than females. While in a review Collishaw et al., (2007) clearly declared that resilience was not a function of gender. Jaffee, Caspi, Moffitt, Polo-Tomas, and Taylor (2007) posited that males and females were equally likely to be resilient and individual strengths played a more important role in distinguishing resilient from non-resilient males rather than females. In the study by Sun and Stewart (2007) in the same year also revealed that gender differences in resilience changed over time and suggested that these differences deserve further investigations in view of their potential implications for mental health prevention and promotion.

In numbers of studies there are mixed finding also regarding gender differences. In some studies males have been reported more resilient than female and the vice-versa.

In few studies there have been no gender differences as such. Ebrahimi Dehghani and others (2012) also reported that there is no meaningful resiliency difference regarding resilience between male and female students. Igdorural youths, Chukwuoji and Ajaero (2014) reported no significant difference on resilience among male and female student. A recent study done by Sreehari and Nair (2015) suggested that no gender differences in resilience among adolescents, while on the other hand, Kamble (2015) found significant gender differences on resilience. However, Evidence of gendered psychological resources (e.g., agency, mastery and worth) in favour of males which may provide the requisite foundation to enable resilience characteristics. The work of Shanahan and Hofer (2005) has been supported by earlier studies showing higher resilience in adolescent males as compared to females (Campbell-Sills et al., 2009; von Soest et al., 2010; Waktaar and Torgersen, 2012; Abukari and Laser, 2013; Stratta et al., 2013; Ying et al., 2014). Among older populations, males had been reported more resilient as compared to their counterparts (Boardman et al., 2008). Similar result found in the Chinese community where men scored higher on resilience than women (Yu &Zhang, 2007).

Thus it was seen that in a numbers of studies there are mixed finding regarding gender differences. The review suggests that even though some high risk students can seem to be resilient in terms of their behavior, while meeting societal expectation or showing competence, many of these same students might still struggle with inner distress in the form of problems such as depression and anxiety.

Studies Related to Personality and Mental Health

Many studies affirmed that five-factor personality traits related to mental health such as Goodwin and Friedman (2006) investigated on health status and five-factor personality traits among adults in the United States. Their results showed that higher level of conscientiousness was associated with reducing level of mental and physical disorders while a higher level of neuroticism was significantly contributed to increase in mental disorders.

Recently a study was conducted by Zarei, Zeinalipour, Sough, Adli, and Sough (2013) on personality traits and general health among students. They explored a positive and significant relationship between personality traits of extraversion, openness (flexibility), agreeableness, conscientiousness and general health, while a negative relationship was found between neuroticism and general health. Further, they also demonstrated that neuroticism predicts 0.45 % of the variance of general health among students. Researches are also showing that there is a significant relationship between personality traits and mental health (Haren et al., 2003; Hayas et al., 2002).

Personality is also associated with various health behaviors as they contribute in some way to decide about lifestyle behaviors. For example, highly extroverted individuals were more likely to smoke cigarettes, consume alcohol, binge drink, and have multiple sexual partners (Raynor & Levine, 2009). Highly conscientious individuals were more likely to wear seat belts, utilize alcohol-related harm reduction, exercise, get enough sleep, and consume fruits and vegetables. They were also less likely to smoke cigarettes, consume alcohol, and binge drink. Another study showed that highly conscientious individuals were also less likely to engage in risky behaviors and were more likely to engage in healthy behaviors (Bogg & Roberts, 2004).

In a study Shirazi, Khan and Ansari (2002) examined the relationship between mental health and personality characteristics of students. A total of 300 participants were randomly selected from Aligarh Muslim University, Aligarh, India. The result shows that there is a significant correlation between mental health and personality characteristics. The result of multiple regression analysis using the stepwise method found agreeableness, neuroticism, and openness as the significant predictors of mental health. Finally, independent t-test found no significant difference in the mean scores of professional and non-professional students' mental health and personality characteristics in terms of gender.

Sadeghi, Ofoghi and Azizi (2015) from University of Guilan examined the relationship between196 students' (Faculty of Humanities) personality characteristics and mental health. Results showed that there was a strong relationship between personality characteristics of neurotic, openness, extraversion and being conscionable with mental health. Also, there were no significant differences among students with respect to different courses but significant difference with respect to gender and age. In another study Shaheen, Jahan, and Shaheen (2014) investigated the role of self-esteem in development of aggression among adolescents.100 male and 100 female students were selected from senior secondary school of Aligarh Muslim University Aligarh. Result showed that there was significant negative correlation between self - esteem and aggression. In gender differences, it was found that male students scored significantly higher on self esteem in comparison to female students. It was also explored that male students scored significantly higher on different dimensions of aggression (i.e. physical, verbal, anger and hostility) in comparison to female students. Another study reported an association between the personality traits viz., agreeableness, openness and subjective well-being (Haslam & Bastian, 2009). The positive relationship indicated that an increase in neuroticism could lead to an unhealthy mental health outcome. This result is consistent with the past research findings (Yang, Chiu, Soong & Chen, 2008) which revealed that neuroticism can be associated with a single episode of a depressive symptom and on extroversion and conscientiousness. These finding also contradicts with the work of (Wismeijer & Assen, 2008) indicated that extraversion and conscientiousness are associated with subjective well-being among students of university. In addition to that interaction between levels of family conflict and personality traits also helps to explain the differences in mental health outcome (Tan, 2007).

In a recent study Cheng, Weiss and Siegel (2015) examined the relative contributions of individual characteristics of personality and health behaviors to subjective well-being among university-attending emerging young adults. Three dimensions of well-being were assessed i.e., effective (positive affect), physical/mental (overall health), and cognitive (quality of life). The sample (N=599) consisted of students of various racial/ethnic backgrounds, including white/non-Hispanic, Hispanic/Latino, Asian/Pacific Islander, and Black/African, American from a large public university in Southern California. Respondents completed the student health survey which consisted of items on basic demographics, substance use, health behaviors, affect balance scale, extraversion and neuroticism subscales of the Big Five taxonomy of personality, quality of life scale, and an online food-intake survey for seven days. Extraverted individuals reported more positive affect and higher quality of life. Neuroticism was associated with the less positive effect, poorer health, and lower quality of life. Findings indicate that health behaviors are the important correlates of three dimensions of well-being over and above the effects of personality traits.

In the same year Mobarakeh, Juhari, Yaacob, Redzuan, and Mobarakeh (2015) reported the study to determine the relationship between locus of control and psychological well-being among Iranian adolescent migrants in Kuala-Lumpur, Malaysia. The participants were 300 Iranian student adolescents that comprise (143 male, and 157 female) in the age range of 13-16 years. The results showed that there was a significant relationship between locus of control and adolescent's psychological well-being. Internal locus of control was positively associated with psychological well-being, while external locus of control was negatively associated with psychological well-being. In this connection a meta-analysis study was done and it was found that level of neuroticism has been emerged to be the best predictor of life satisfaction and happiness (De Neve & Cooper, 1998). In an extensive review of the study also reported that conscientiousness-related traits were negatively related to all risky health-related behaviors and positively related to all beneficial health-related behaviors (Bogg & Roberts, 2004). This study demonstrates the importance of conscientiousness' contribution to the health process through its relationship to health-related behaviors. It is now well-established that conscientiousness predicts health and longevity in various populations and over long periods of time (Kern & Friedman, 2008; Roberts et al., 2007).Conscientious children and adolescents usually grow up to smoke less, eat healthier foods, wear seatbelts, and engage in a range of other healthy behaviors (Bogg & Roberts, 2004; Lodi-Smith et al., 2010).

Thus, it was observed in a number of studies that personality and mental health reveals a positive relationship. In consideration of mental health-related problems, it can be concluded that personality traits have important role to play in both physical and psychological consequences. Because of such traits i.e., anger and tension, people expect to have coronary illnesses and to have higher blood pressure. In addition, they are more inclined to depression, chronic stress, sleeping disorders and anxiety due to their psychological characteristics. The above studies confirm that there exist positive relationship between personality and mental health.

Studies Related to Gender Difference and Personality Traits

Many studies have demonstrated conflicting results regarding gender difference in adolescents' personality trait. In a study Costa, Terracciano, and McCrae (2001) examined the gender differences in personality traits across cultures with Revised NEO Personality Inventory. 26 cultures suggested that gender differences are small relative to individual's variation within genders; differences are replicated across cultures for both college-aged and adult samples, and differences are broadly consistent with gender stereotypes. Adolescents' girls were reported higher in neuroticism, agreeableness, warmth, and openness to feelings, whereas adolescent boys were higher in assertiveness and openness to ideas. Contrary to predictions from evolutionary theory, the magnitude of gender differences varied across cultures.

In another study Costa, McCrae, and Martin (2008) found that young adolescent girls were higher in extraversion and openness as compared to boys. Similar results also described by McCrae, Costa, et al., (2005) and McCrae et al.,

(2002), whereas Branje, Van Lieshout, and Gerris (2007) reported contradictory findings that boys tended to be more extroverted and open to experience than girls. McCrae and colleagues (2002) revealed higher levels of agreeableness and neuroticism in girls. A similar finding was revealed by Klimstra, Hale, Raaijmakers, Branje, and Meeus (2009), whereas Branje et al. (2007) have demonstrated no gender differences on these two dimensions i.e., agreeableness and neuroticism. However Klimstra and colleagues (2009) have suggested that these inconsistencies might be explained by differences in populations or cultures sampled or by variations in the particular adolescent age groups selected.

Goodwin and Gotlib (2004) examined to determine the association between gender and the Big Five personality factors, and identified the role of personality factors in the association between gender and depression among adults in the United States. Data were drawn from the Midlife Development in the United States Survey. Analyses were conducted to examine the relationship between gender and depression, and to test whether this association is moderated by neuroticism. Levels of neuroticism, agreeableness, extraversion, and conscientiousness were significantly higher among females as compared to males. In contrast, level of openness to experience found significantly higher in males. Female were associated with increased odds of experiencing depression. Results showed that neuroticism played a significant contributory role in the relationship between being female and major depression, though the role of gender remained statistically significant. These data suggest that gender differences in personality factors, specificaly neuroticism may play a key role in gender differences in depression.

Benjamin, Chapman, Duberstein, Sorensen, and Jeffey (2007) examined gender differences in a sample of 486 older adults, ranged from 65-98years using the NEO-Five Factor Inventory. Mean and Covariance Structure models testing gender differences at the level of latent traits revealed higher levels of neuroticism and agreeableness in older women as compared to older men. The consistency of these findings was observed with prior work in younger samples attests to the stability of gender differentiation in neuroticism and agreeableness across the lifespan. Gender differences in these traits have been considered in personality research among older adults as well as middle age and younger adults. In further review Weisberg, De Young and Hirsh (2011) also explored gender differences in personality traits, both at the level of the Big Five and at the sub level of two aspects within each Big Five domain. Replicating previous findings, women reported higher in big five extraversion, agreeableness, and neuroticism scores than men. However, more extensive gender differences were found at the level of the aspects with significant gender differences appearing in both aspects of every Big Five trait. For extraversion, openness to experience, and conscientiousness, the gender differences were found to be diverged at the expected level, rendering them either small or undetectable at the Big Five level. These findings clarify the nature of gender differences in personality and highlight the utility of measuring personality. In a very recent Study Sharma and Gulati (2015) also reported that males have scored significantly higher on psychoticism, whereas, females were significantly more on extraversion. Neuroticism dimension was nearly equal in both males and females.

In numbers of studies there are mixed finding regarding gender differences in different personality traits. In some studies males have been reported significant differences in different personality dimension than female and the vice-versa.

Studies Related to Spiritual Intelligence, Resilience, Personality and Mental Health

In a very recent review by Kumari, Joshi, and Singh. (2015) concluded that spiritual intelligence and mental health have positive relationship. They also reported that one of the important reasons could be that spirituality provides a number of psychological benefits to individual by offering people a sense of purpose and meaning of life.

Sood and Bakhshi (2013) indicated in their study that resilience was positively associated with all the dimensions of spiritual intelligence. The positive relationship also exists between resilience and mental health. Regression analysis indicates that resilience and spiritual intelligence meaningfully explain mental health. Resilience has more significant role in predicting and explaining mental health. Some of the dimensions of spiritual Intelligence too have a significant role in explaining mental health. Shabani, Hassan, Ahmad & Baba (2011) studied that spiritual intelligence and emotional intelligence can be considered as an important predictor for mental health. The result demonstrated that mental health can be influenced by spiritual intelligence and emotional intelligence. In addition, the moderating effect of gender on the relationship of spiritual intelligence and emotional intelligence with mental health was not established.

In a study Ebrahimi, Dehghani, and Uavadan (2012) indicated that there was a positively meaningful relationship between resiliency and mental health, and also between spiritual intelligence and resiliency. Results of multiple regressions analysis indicated that mental health and spiritual intelligence meaningfully explain resiliency. Mental health has a more significant role in predicting and explaining resiliency. Due to the fact that people with higher resiliency represent a higher degree of mental health, it could be concluded that providing vital factors (religion and spirit) to enhance resiliency can strengthen people in the face of mental stresses, tension, and depression.

In a study, Hamid, Keikhosravani, Babamiri, and Dehghani (2012) investigated the relationship between mental health, spiritual intelligence, and resiliency among the Kermanshah Medical Science University. The results indicated that there was a positive relationship between mental health and resiliency. Also, there was a positive relationship between spiritual intelligence and resiliency. The results of multiple regressions showed that the mental health had a strong role to predict resiliency. They also concluded that mental health and spiritual intelligence had a significant role to predict resiliency.

In a recent study Shi, Liu, Wang, and Wang (2015) examined the correlations among anxiety, big five personality traits, and resilience. Result revealed the four traits viz., extraversion, agreeableness, conscientiousness, and openness to experience were negatively related to anxiety symptoms whereas neuroticism was positively related to anxiety symptoms. The results also demonstrated that extraversion, agreeableness, conscientiousness, and openness were positively related to resilience while neuroticism was negatively related to it. Specifically, agreeableness, openness, and conscientiousness were all negatively associated with anxiety symptoms whereas neuroticism was positively associated with the symptoms.

Fayombo (2010) also investigated the relationships between the big five personality traits i.e., conscientiousness, agreeableness, neuroticism, openness to experience, extraversion and psychological resilience among 397 Caribbean secondary school adolescents. Results revealed significant positive relationships between the personality traits i.e., conscientiousness, agreeableness, openness to experience, extraversion and psychological resilience, while neuroticism was negatively correlated with psychological resilience.

Green and Noble (2010) demostrated that college and university students are curious to explore the questions regarding spirituality through higher education. This study also reveals the intellectual and personal effects of this approach for undergraduate students about consciousness. Results showed that students were more open to diverse ideas about consciousness, self-aware, and more committed to meditation and self-reflection.

Majority of studies in this area have been shown positive but few studies show mixed findings. In a study Amrai, Farahani, Ebrahimi, and Bagherian (2011) examined the relationship between personality traits and spiritual intelligence among university students. In this correlation research, 205 students of University of Tehran were chosen using multiple cluster sampling. Findings showed that there was a negative relation between neuroticism and spiritual intelligence and positive relation between conscientiousness, agreeableness, and extroversion accordingly. Openness to experience had no relation with spiritual intelligence.

Beshlideh, Charkhabi, Kalkhoran, and Marashi (2011) expanded the evidence relating to spiritual intelligence by determining whether the big five personality traits can predict spiritual intelligence. Further, the goal was to find out the direction of the prediction. 270 male graduate students of Shahid Chamran University at Ahvaz were selected using the simple random sampling. Results showed that the three personality traits viz., extraversion, agreeableness, and conscientiousness have significant correlations with spiritual intelligence. It was further concluded that the students with extraversion, agreeableness and conscientiousness, features are more likely to have higher spiritual intelligence while people with higher openness necessarily do not have higher spiritual intelligence.

Farsani, Arofzad, and Hosaini (2013) also examined the relationship between spiritual intelligence with personality traits among physical education managers in Isfahan province. Results showed that there was a positive and meaningful correlation between spiritual intelligence and dimensions of personality i.e., openness to experience, conscientiousness, agreeableness, and extraversion. On the other hand, results indicated the negative and significant correlation between neuroticism and spiritual intelligence sub-scales. It was concluded that the spiritual intelligence and personality traits are two important components for physical education managers and there was meaningful role in the organization.

In a study Lockenhoff, Ironson, O'Cleirigh, and Costa (2009) explored the association between five-factor personality domains and facets and spirituality/ religiousness as well as their joint association with mental health in a diverse sample of people living with HIV (aged 18–66 year). Spirituality/religiousness showed stronger associations with conscientiousness, openness to experience, and agreeableness than with neuroticism and extraversion. Both personality traits and spirituality/religiousness were significantly linked to mental health. Personality traits explained unique variance in mental health above spirituality and religiousness.

Further, the preceding review also suggests that all the affected related variables should be assumed to have a direct effect on the mental health and some of them may also have an indirect effect on mental health. Today the field of psychology has shown the tendency towards the spiritual dimension and wide horizon for extended research has spread, that can reflect the profound influence of spiritual force on the human body and mind and makes clear the importance of spiritual intelligence. Spiritual intelligence and resilience were found to mediate some of the links between personality and mental health of adolescents. These findings suggest that underlying spiritual intelligence, resilience and personality traits contribute to the beneficial effects on mental health of adolescents.

Thus, the present study aims at exploring the relationship between spiritual intelligence, resilience and personality in context to mental health of adolescents.

Rationale of the study

The present study takes into account the gap and makes an attempt to examine the role spiritual intelligence, resilience and personality in the mental health of adolescents and to explores how and to what extent the various variables relate, affect and contribute to our understanding of this relationship.

1. Growing literature is available on the association between spiritual intelligence, resilience and mental health but researches regarding spiritual intelligence and the personality areas are still neglected, so the present investigation made an attempt to understand these concepts more vividly.

2. After an exhaustive review of the literature, it was discovered that very few studies have been conducted on spiritual intelligence and some dimensions of personality traits i.e. agreeableness, conscientiousness, and extraversion which have shown positive results but the researches on personality dimension with special reference to openness to experience and spiritual intelligence are very few and have shown mixed results.

3. Although the literature related to spiritual intelligence, resilience, personality and mental health of adolescents in the western world is available but it is still lacking in Indian context. Thus, it needs to be examined in Indian context.

4. In addition, there are mixed findings related to gender differences in spiritual intelligence, resilience and personality.

5. Not only the role of spiritual intelligence, resilience, personality and mental health have been investigated in the present research but also an attempt has been made to understand the inter-relationship between the said variables.

6. The adolescence period is the best time to develop positive emotions and training skills because adolescents seek to find their identity and future personality in this period. Spiritual intelligence has a significant influence on the life of adolescent and it goes without saying that adolescence is a sensitive period which requires specific training to make a brighter future. Therefore, research in this area particularly on adolescents' sample could make a major contribution.

7. In the context of mental health, resilience can be viewed as the ability to handle stress positively. Adolescents' stress can come from multiple directions e.g., school, relationships (with friends, romantic partners, and parents), hormonal and physical changes, impending decisions about college and career, pressures to conform or to engage in risky behaviors, family financial problems, dangerous neighborhoods etc. A unique aspect of this study is that all the domains of resilience have been examined together.

8. The study of personality in various forms can point out the ways in which personality constructs can be used to promote adolescents and emerging adult wellness, to help prevent or reduce risk-taking behavior, and to facilitate successful transitions into responsible adulthood among today's youth. The relative importance of this variable has its own contribution in the study.

9. The study is significant and important in recognizing the factors influencing adolescent's mental health which can motivate the students for the right direction & identify those students who need assistance to achieve the desired goal in future. Certain variables like resilience, spiritual intelligence are still an exploratory state. Thus research is required to clarify the extent and the mean by which these variables influence the mental health.

Thus the present study aims at studying the role of spiritual intelligence, resilience and personality in mental health of adolescents.

Operational definition of the variables -

Spiritual intelligence-It is concerned with the inner life of mind and spirit and its relationship to being in the world.

Resilience- It refers to an individual's ability to cope with stress and adversity whether outcomes are successfully or not is determined by the presence (and bounce back) of both risk factors and protective factors over time.

Personality- It refers to the different facets of individual traits and their unique adjustment with their environment.

Mental health- It is a psychological state of someone who is functioning at a satisfactory level of emotion and behavioral adjustment.

OBJECTIVES

Incorporating above mentioned gap in literature and considered potential importance of variables included in the present study, the following objectives were prepared.

1. To examine the relationship between spiritual intelligence and mental health of adolescents.
2. To examine the relationship between resilience and mental health of adolescents.
3. To examine the relationship between personality and mental health of adolescents.
4. To examine the gender differences in spiritual intelligence, resilience, and personality.
5. To verify the contribution of spiritual Intelligence, resilience, and personality in the prediction of mental health of adolescents and relative importance of these variables.

HYPOTHESES

Based on prior finding and theoretical background the following hypotheses were framed on the basis of research objectives.

H1: Spiritual intelligence would be positively correlated with mental health of adolescents.

H2: Resilience would be positively correlated with mental health of adolescents.

H3 (a): Neuroticism dimension of personality would be negatively correlated with mental health of adolescents.

(b): Extraversion dimension of personality would be positively correlated with mental health of adolescents.

(c): Openness to experience dimension of personality would be positively correlated with mental health of adolescents

(d): Agreeableness dimension of personality would be positively correlated with mental health of adolescents.

(e): Conscientiousness dimension of personality would be positively correlated with mental health of adolescents.

H4 (a): Spiritual intelligence would be higher in boys as compared to girls.

(b): Resilience would be higher in boys as compared to girls.

(c): Girls would score higher on neuroticism as compared to boys.

(d): Boys would score higher on extraversion, agreeableness, and conscientiousness as compared to girls.

(e): Boys would score higher on openness to experience as compared to girls.

H5: Spiritual intelligence, resilience, and personality would significantly predict the mental health of adolescents.

CHAPTER- III

METHODOLOGY

This chapter deals with the methodological and procedural aspects of the problem. It explains the operational definitions, design followed in the selection of the sample, hypotheses, description of tools and procedure adopted in data collection, and data analyses.

In the present research work, an attempt has been made to examine the role of spiritual intelligence, resilience, and personality in the mental health of adolescents. The present study follows a correlational design in which spiritual intelligence, resilience, and personality were treated as the predictor variables and mental health was treated as the criterion variable.

Design

In the present study, an attempt has been made to examine the relationship of spiritual intelligence, resilience, personality and mental health of adolescents. The present study follows a correlational design. Spiritual intelligence, resilience and personality have been treated as predictors and mental health as criterion variable among adolescents. Hence in order to obtained detailed information from a relatively large number of cases, the most suitable method i.e. simple descriptive survey was used.

Sample

The present research study was conducted on a sample of 400 students (200 male and 200 female) aged 17 to 19 years. The students were selected from different schools of Varanasi city.

Profile of Participants-Gender wise (N=400)

Gender	No. of Participants	Percentage
Male	200	50
Female	200	50
Total	**400**	**100 %**

Depicts the percentage of the total sample size of 400 out of which 200 (50%) were male and 200 (50%) were females.

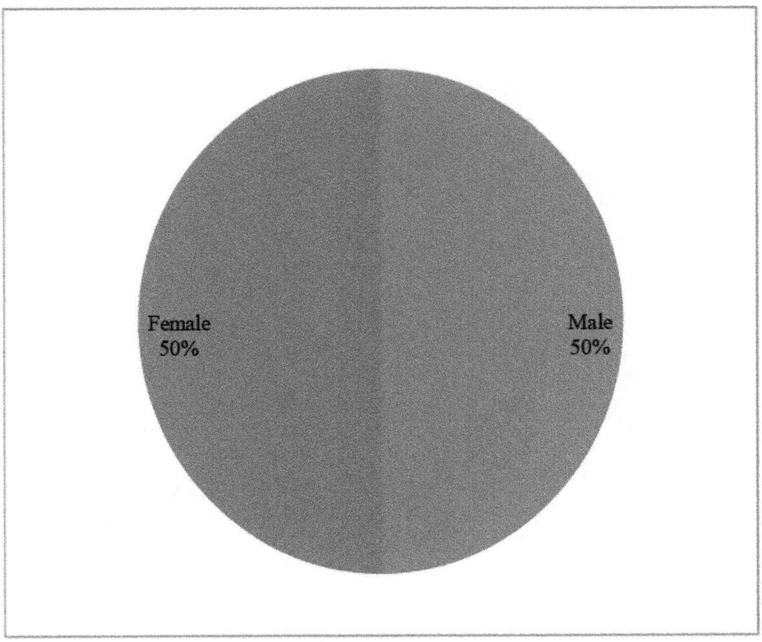

Pie chart representation of participants (gender wise).

Profile of Participants-Age (N=400)

Age	No. of Participants	Percentage
17 years	199	49.80
18 years	138	34.50
19 years	63	15.80
Total	**400**	**100%**

Depicts age wise percentage of participants selected for study. The proportion of total sample of participants aged 17 years was 49.80% (N=199), 18 years was 34.50% (N=138) and 19 years was 15.80% age range 17 to 19 years.

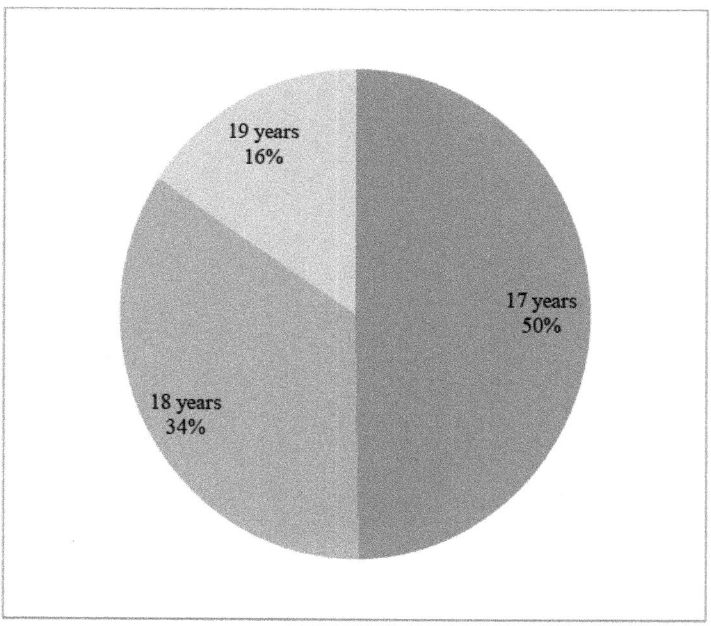

Pie chart representation of participant's age.

Profile of Participants-Family Structure (N=400)

Family Structure	No. of Participants	Percent
Nuclear Family	170	42.50
Joint Family	230	57.50
Total	**400**	**100%**

Depicts percentage value of the 400 participants. The proportion of total sample of participants residing nuclear family was 42.50% (N=170) and joint family was 57.50% (N=230).

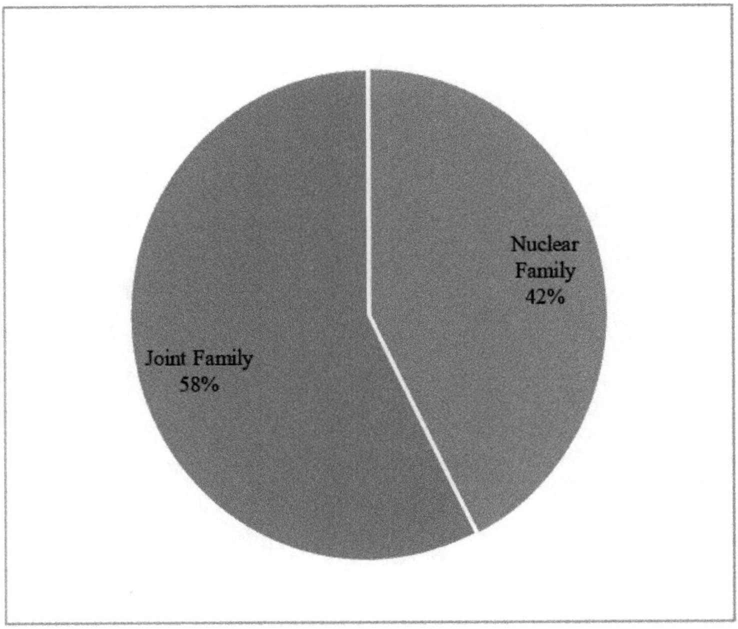

Pie chart representation of participant's family structure.

Profile of Participants- Parents' Occupation (N=400)

Parents' Occupation	No. of Participants	Percent
Govt. Service	101	25.30
Pvt. Service	8	2.00
Business	291	72.80
Total	**400**	**100%**

Depicts percentage value of 400 participants selected for the study. The proportion of total sample of participants's parents 101(25.30%) were in government service, 8 (2.00%) were in private service and 291(72.80%) participants had their business.

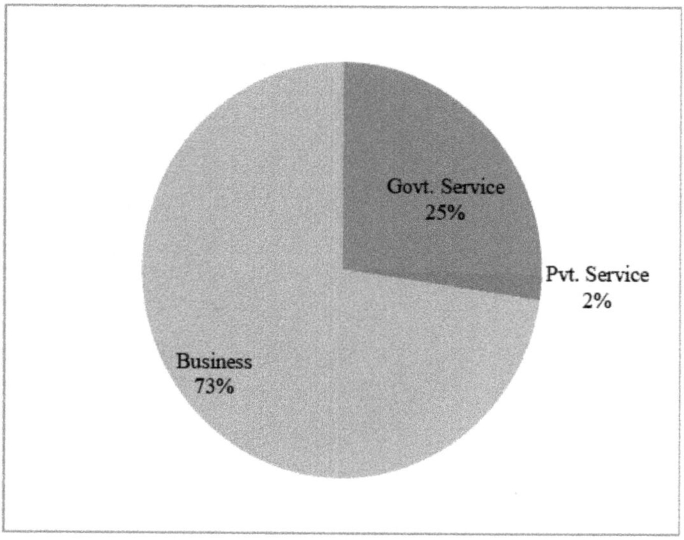

Pie chart representation of participant's parents' Occupation.

Measures

The selection of suitable tools is of vital importance for successful research. The success of any research endeavor is largely dependent upon the tools which are used for data collection. It is essential that the tool itself should be well standardized, reliable and valid. Secondly, they should be suitable for the chosen sample. To study the variables in the present investigation the following psychometrics devices were utilized.

1. Personal Data Blank
2. Mental Health Inventory
3. Resilience Scale
4. Personality Inventory (NEO-FFI)
5. King's Spiritual intelligence scale

Personal Data Blank

In order to obtain relevant personal information about the respondent included in the sample, a personal data sheet (in Hindi) was designed by the researcher. Information related to name, age, gender, caste, sex, residential background, address, birth order, and type of family etc were included in the sheet. They were instructed to fill this sheet before the completion of all four standardized tests.

Mental Health Inventory (M.H.I)

Mental Health Inventory (M.H.I.) developed by Jagdish & A.K. Srivastava (1996) was used for measuring mental health of individuals in various sphere of life and has been designed to measure mental health (positive) of normal individuals. The Mental Health Inventory consists of 56 items and six popular indices i.e. positive self-evaluation (PSE), perception of reality (PR), integration of personality (IP), autonomy (AUTNY), group-oriented attitudes (GOA), and environmental mastery (EM). Brief descriptions of each of these indices are given below.

Positive Self-Evaluation (PSE): It includes self-confidence, self-acceptance, self-identity, feeling of worthwhileness, the realization of one's potentialities, etc.

Perception of Reality (PR): It is related to perception free from need distortion, the absence of excessive fantasy and a broad outlook on the world.

Integration of Personality (IP): It indicates the balance of psychic forces in the individual and includes the ability to understand and to share other people's emotions, the ability to concentrate at work and interest in several activities.

Autonomy (AUTNY): It includes a stable set of internal standards for one's action, dependence upon own potentialities rather than dependence on other people.

Group-Oriented Attitudes (GOA): It is associated with the ability to get along with others, work with others and ability to find recreation.

Environmental Mastery (EM): It includes efficiency in meeting situational requirements, the ability to work and play the ability to take responsibilities and capacity for adjustment.

Reliability:

The reliability of the inventory was determined by 'split-half method' using the odd-even procedure. The table gives the reliability coefficients of different and overall dimensions of mental health.

Sl.No.	Dimensions of M.H.	Reliability Index
1.	Positive Self-Evaluation	0.75
2.	Perception of Reality	0.71
3.	Integration of Personality	0.72
4.	Autonomy	0.72
5.	Group-Oriented Attitudes	0.74
6.	Environmental Mastery	0.71
	Overall	**0.73**

Validity:

Construct validity of the inventory was determined by finding the coefficient of correlation between scores on Mental Health Inventory and General Health Questionnaire (Gold berg, 1978). It was found to be 0.54 and with Personal Adjustment (a sub-scale of S.D. Inventory) developed by Pestonjee (1973) was 0.57.

Scoring:

In the present scale, 4 alternative responses have been assigned to each statement i.e. always, often, rarely and never. 4 scores for to 'always', 3 scores to 'Often', 2, scores to 'Rarely', and 1, scores to 'Never' respectively.

Resilience Scale

The Resilience Scale originally developed by Mampane (2005) was used for the purpose of identifying resilient and non-resilient adolescents. The scale consists of 25 items based on the following resilience factors: Commitment, future aspirations, problem-solving, role models, self-awareness, sense of control and support. The statements are short, simple and easy to understand and reflect descriptions of behaviors that relate to activities, events and characteristics assumed relevant and applicable to an adolescent's life.

Reliability:

The reliability of this scale was established at an alpha value 0.82.

Scoring:

The Questionnaire consists of 25 items. The responses were to marked on a scale of 4 to 1, ranging from 'strongly agree' to 'strongly disagree'. A higher score indicates higher resilience.

Personality Scale

NEO-FFI- Personality traits of adolescents was measured by the NEO Five-Factor Inventory (NEO-FFI), which was originally developed by Costa and Mc Care in 1992. The NEO-FFI is a well recognized, extensively tested and widely used scale to measure the Big Five Personality dimensions (e.g. Mooradian & Olver, 1997; Renner, 2002). This inventory consists of sixty items (twelve items for each factor) and based on five-point Likert format (from "strongly agree" to "strongly disagree").

Reliability:

Reliability (Cronbach's Alpha) was found to be 0.85 for neuroticism, 0.80 for extraversion, 0.75 for agreeableness, 0.83 for conscientiousness factor and 0.66 for openness.

Scoring:

The participants responded to each item on a 5-point scale anchored with strongly disagree (0) and strongly agree (4). The twelve items for each domain are added together to provide a total score for that personality domain. Higher scores represent more characteristics of that domain.

King's Spiritual intelligence scale:

The spiritual intelligence self-report questionnaire developed by King (2008) was used for measurement of spiritual intelligence. This Spiritual intelligence scale consists of 24 items and four indices i.e. existential thinking, transcendental awareness, personal meaning production, and conscious state expansion. Brief descriptions of each of these indices are given below:

Critical Existential Thinking

The capacity to critically contemplate the nature of existence, reality, the universe, space, time, and other existential/metaphysical issues, the capacity to contemplate non-existential issues in relation to one's existence i.e., from existential perspective.

Perspective Meaning Production

The ability to derive personal meaning and purpose from all physical and mental experiences, including the capacity to create and master a life purpose.

Transcendental Awareness

The capacity to identify transcendent dimension patterns of the self i.e., a transpersonal or transcendent self, of others, and of the physical world e.g., nonmaterialism during normal states of consciousness, accompanied by the capacity to their relationship to one's self and to the physical.

Conscious State Expansion

The ability to enter and exit higher states of consciousness e.g. pure consciousness, cosmic, consciousness, unity, oneness and other states of trance at one's own discretion (as in deep contemplation, meditation, prayer, etc).

Reliability

The reliability of this inventory was determined by 'split-half method' using the odd-even procedure. The table gives the reliability coefficients of different dimensions of spiritual intelligence.

Sr. No.	Dimensions of S.I.	Reliability Index
1.	Critical Existential Thinking	0.88
2.	Perspective Meaning Production	0.87
3.	Transcendental Awareness	0.89
4.	Conscious State Expansion	0.94
	Overall	**0.95**

Scoring

David B. King (2008) constructed the Spiritual Intelligence Self- Report Inventory (SISRI 24) on the basis of Likert scale. The positive statements were given the following weights i.e., not at all true of me, not very true of me, somewhat true of me, very true of me and completely true of me.

Negative statements were scored vice-versa. All the statements were positive except statement no.6 (negative statement). The scoring of the test was done according to the instructions provided in the respective manual.

Hindi adaptation of all questionnaires was done by the researcher during the course of study.

Procedure

The investigator contacted the principals of the selected institutions and received permission for data collection. After making adequate sitting arrangements, the investigator established proper rapport with the respondents. Then test booklets were distributed and purpose of the testing was stated in brief. Assurance was given for maintaining strict confidentiality of the information given by them. The data was collected randomly from the respondents from different schools of Varanasi city. First of all personal data bank was given to the each respondent. After that SISRI-24, NEO-FFI, Resilience and Mental Health Inventory were administered to the participants. As they completed responses on given measures, data was collected and they were thanked for participation. Scoring of data was done and data was analyzed according to defined rules according to the instructions given in the manuals.

Scoring and tabulation

The entire booklets were scored according to the dimensions mentioned in their respective manuals with the help of scoring keys by the investigator himself. Incomplete booklets were excluded from scoring and tabulation. Raw scores were entered carefully. Further, the data was computerized for different statistical analysis.

Data Analyses

The obtained raw scores on different scales were entered in the computer. To test the gender differences among adolescents on spiritual intelligence, resilience, and personality t-ratio was calculated. Then to test the relationship between spiritual intelligence, resilience, personality and mental health Pearson correlation was calculated.

Hierarchical regression analyses and hierarchical stepwise regression analyses were performed to test whether predictor variables (spiritual intelligence, resilience, and personality) significant predict the mental health of adolescents.

The present chapter was aimed at explaining the statement of the problem; the methodology, measures, procedure and data analysis. In the next chapter, the results of the present work will be presented.

CHAPTER- IV

RESULTS

The present chapter embodies the results obtained from the computerized statistical analyses of responses of the subjects on four different psychometric devices. The statistics applied includes the computation of means, standard deviation, correlation coefficient (Pearson's r and multiple regression analysis. The chapter reports the findings from the statistical analyses as they relate to the research question. A summary of the findings will conclude the chapter. The scores for the analysis were obtained on the basis of the responses of the subjects from different schools of Varanasi on four different psychometric tools viz., spiritual intelligence, resilience, personality and mental health along with personal data blank. The responses were entered into SPSS-20 software for analyses.

To test the hypothesis formulated for the present study that spiritual intelligence has a positive relationship with mental health correlational analysis was performed. The result of the correlational analysis is displayed in Table 1.

Table 1: Summary of correlation analysis between demographic variables, all the predictors (spiritual intelligence, resilience, and personality) and criterion (mental health) variables.

Variables	Spiritual intelligence	Resilience	Openness to experience	Conscientio-usness	Extraversion	Agreeableness	Neuroticism	Mental health
Age	-.069	.106*	-.025	.160**	.073	.074	-.032	-.048
Gender	.012	-.339**	-.142**	-.348**	-.455**	-.368**	.148**	-.590**
Family Structure	-.040	-.040	.123*	-.067	.051	-.044	.036	.140**
Parent Occupation	.078	.053	.051	-.010	-.013	.068	.010	.053

** P<0.01, *P<0.05

Table 1 shows the result of correlational analysis revealed that age was significantly positively correlated with resilience (r= 0.106, p<0.05), and conscientiousness (r= 0.160, p<0.01), whereas age was positively correlated with extraversion (r= 0.073) and agreeableness (r= 0.074) and negatively correlated with spiritual intelligence (r= -0.044), openness to experience (r= -0.025), neuroticism (r= -0.032), and over all mental health (r= -0.048) but it was not statistically significant.

Gender was positively correlated with spiritual intelligence (r= 0.12) but it was not significant, and neuroticism (r= 0.148, p<0.01) was significantly positively correlated with spiritual intelligence. Whereas, gender was significantly negatively correlated with resilience (r= -0.339, p<0.001), openness to experience (r= - 0.142, p<0.001), conscientiousness (r= -0.348, p<0.001) extraversion (r= -0.455, p<0.001), agreeableness (r= -0.368, p<0.001) and mental health (r= -0.590, p<0.001).

Family structure was significantly positively correlated with openness to experience (r= 0.123, p<0.005) and over all mental health (r= 0.140, p<0.001). Family structure was also positively correlated with extraversion (r= 0.051) and neuroticism (r= 0.036) and negatively correlated with spiritual intelligence (r= -0.040), resilience (r= - 0.040), conscientiousness (r= -0.067), and agreeableness (r= -0.044) but it was not significant.

Parent's occupation was not correlated with spiritual intelligence (r= 0.078), resilience (r=0.053), openness to experience (r=0.051), conscientiousness (r= - 0.010), extraversion (r= -0.013), agreeableness (r= 0.068), neuroticism (r= 0.010) and over all mental health (r= 0.053).

Table 2: Summary of correlation analyses between all the dimensions of spiritual intelligence and mental health of adolescents

MH / SI	Positive Self Evaluation	Perception of Reality	Integration of Personality	Autonomy	Group-Oriented Attitude	Environmental Mastery	Mental Health
Critical Existence Thinking	.134**	.097	.175**	.059	.165**	.028	.190**
Personal Meaning Production	.150**	.036	.084	.093	.017	.050	.119*
Transcendent Awareness	.422**	.174**	.188**	.227**	.147**	.192**	.373**
Conscious State Expansion	-.431**	-.266**	-.303**	-.384**	-.391**	-.200**	-.541**
Spiritual Intelligence	.366**	.187**	.233**	.224**	.172**	.168**	.374**

**p<0.01, *p<0.05

Table 2 shows the results of correlational analysis of all the dimensions of spiritual intelligence and mental health. Critical existence thinking dimension of spiritual intelligence was significantly positively correlated with positive self-evaluation (r=0.134, P<0.01), integration of personality (r=0.175, p<0.01), group-oriented attitude (r=0.165, p<0.01) and overall mental health (r=0.190, p<0.01). Although the direction of the relationship of critical existence thinking with the perception of reality (r=0.097), autonomy (r=0.059) and environmental mastery (r=0.028) was positive but it was not significant.

Personal meaning production dimension of spiritual intelligence was significantly positively correlated with positive self-evaluation (r=0.150, p<0.01) and mental health (r=0.119, p<0.05). However, the direction of the relationship of personal meaning production with the perception of reality (r=0.036), integration of personality (r=0.084), autonomy (r=0.093), group-oriented attitude (r=0.017) and environmental mastery (r=0.050) was positive but it was not significant.

Transcendent awareness dimension of spiritual intelligence was significantly positively correlated with all six dimensions of mental health i.e., positive self-evaluation (r=0.422, p<0.01), perception of reality (r=0.174, p<0.01), integration of personality (r=0.188, p<0.01), autonomy (r=0.227, p<0.01), group oriented attitude (r=0.147, p<0.01), environmental mastery (r=0.192, p<0.01) and mental health (r=0.373, P<0.01).

Conscious state expansion dimension of spiritual intelligence was significantly negatively correlated with all six dimensions of mental health i.e., positive self-evaluation (r= -0.431, p<0.01), perception of reality (r= -0.266, p<0.01), integration of personality (r= -0.303, p<0.01), autonomy (r= -0.384, p<0.01), group oriented attitude (r= -0.391, p<0.01), environmental mastery (r= -0.200, p<0.01) and mental health (r= -0.374, p<0.01).

Overall Spiritual Intelligence was significantly positively correlated with all six dimensions of mental health i.e., positive self-evaluation (r=0.366, p<0.01), perception of reality (r=0.187, p<0.01), integration of personality (r=0.233, p<0.01), autonomy (r=0.224, P<0.05), group oriented attitude (r=0.172, p<0.01), environmental mastery (r=0.168, p<0.01) and mental health (r=0.374, p<0.01).

mmary of correlation analyses between all the dimensions of resilience and mental health of adolescents

e	Positive Self Evaluation	Perception Of Reality	Integration of Personality	Autonomy	Group-Oriented Attitude	Environmental Mastery
	-.036	-.078	.020	-.017	-.107*	.003
	.070	.002	.069	.012	-.059	.042
	.060	-.035	.025	-.026	-.084	.089
	.058	.114*	.118*	.151**	-.007	.127*
	.052	.044	.070	.070	.059	.051
	.081	-.015	.109*	.029	.027	.074
	.074	.006	.097	.154**	.033	.149**
	-.338**	-.201**	-.174**	-.154**	-.232**	-.103*
	-.076	-.081	.025	.007	-.151**	.067

01, *p<0.05

The commitment dimension of resilience was negatively correlated with overall mental health, as well as its all dimensions viz., positive self-evaluation (r= -0.036), perception of reality (r= -0.078), and autonomy (r= -0.017) but they are not statistically significant. Only group-oriented attitude (r= -0.107) was significantly negatively correlated with commitment whereas integration of personality (r= 0.020) and environmental mastery (r= 0.003) was positively correlated, but they were also not statistically significant.

Problem solving dimension of resilience was positively correlated with mental health (r=0.041) and its all dimensions viz., positive self-evaluation (r=070), perception of reality (r=0.002), integration of personality (r=0.069), autonomy (r=0.012), and environmental mastery (r=0.042), only group-oriented attitude (r= -0.059) was negatively correlated, but they were not significant.

Support GMSR dimension of resilience was positively correlated with mental health (r= 0.012) and all its dimension viz., positive self-evaluation (r=0.060), integration of personality (r=0.025), and environmental mastery (r= 0.089), whereas perception of reality (r= -0.035), autonomy (r= -0.026), and group oriented attitude (r= -0.084) were negatively associated and they were not significant.

Support HUSR dimension of resilience was significantly positively correlated with perception of reality (r=0.114, $p<0.05$), integration of personality (r=0.118, $p<0.05$), autonomy (r=0.151, $p<0.01$), environmental mastery (r=0.127, $p<0.05$), and overall mental health (r=0.146, $p<0.01$), but positive self-evaluation (r= 0.058) and group oriented attitude (r= -0.007) were negatively correlated and they were not significant.

Role model dimension of resilience was positively correlated with mental health (r= 0.095) and all its dimensions viz., positive self-evaluation (r=0.052), perception of reality (r=0.044), integration of personality (r=0.070), autonomy (r=0.070), group oriented attitude (r=0.059), and environmental mastery (r=0.051), but they were not significant.

Future aspiration dimension of resilience was significantly positively correlated with only integration of personality ($r = 0.110, p < 0.05$), and not significant with positive self evaluation ($r = 0.079$), autonomy ($r = 0.031$), group oriented attitude ($r = 0.021$), environmental mastery ($r = 0.070$), and over all mental health ($r = 0.088$). However, future aspiration dimension was negatively correlated with perception of reality ($r = 0.013$) but it was not significant.

Sense of control dimension of resilience was significantly positively correlated with overall mental health ($r =0.180, p<0.01$) and its two dimensions viz., autonomy ($r = 0.191, p< 0.01$), and environmental mastery ($r = 0.171, p< 0.01$). Although the direction of relationship of sense of control dimension of resilience with positive self-evaluation ($r=0.074$), perception of reality ($r=0.006$), integration of personality ($r=0.097$) and group oriented attitude ($r=0.033$) was positively correlated but it was not significant.

Self-awareness dimension of resilience was significantly negatively correlated with overall mental health ($r= 0-0.336, p<0.001$), and all its dimensions viz., positive self-evaluation ($r = -0.338, p<0.01$), perception of reality ($r= -0.201, p<0.01$), integration of personality ($r= -0.174, p<0.01$), autonomy ($r= -0.154, p<0.01$), group oriented attitude ($r = -0.232, p < 0.01$) and environmental mastery ($r= -0.103, p<0.05$). Over all resilience was negatively correlated with positive self-evaluation ($r= -0.076$), integration of personality ($r= -0.081$), and overall mental health ($r= -0.060$) but it was not significant. Only group oriented attitude dimension of mental health was ($r= -0.151, p<0.001$) significantly negatively correlated. On the other hand, integration of personality ($r=0.025$), autonomy ($r=0.007$), and environmental mastery dimensions of mental health were ($r=0.067$) positively correlated but it was not significant.

Table 4: Summary of correlation analyses between all the dimensions of personality and mental health of adolescents

	Positive Self Evaluation	Perception Of Reality	Integration of Personality	Autonomy	Group-Oriented Attitude	Environmental Mastery	Mental Health
Neuroticism	-.038	.043	.101*	.030	.099*	-.033	.059
Extraversion	.328**	.243**	.200**	.248**	.290**	.231**	.422**
Openness	.265**	.195**	.107*	.119*	.270**	.145**	.306**
Agreeableness	.045	.000	.134**	.119*	-.129**	.121*	.075
Conscientiousness	.016	.009	.076	.055	-.098	.098	.040

**p<0.01, *p<0.05

Table 4 reveals that neuroticism dimension of personality was overall positively correlated with mental health and its two dimensions i.e., perception of reality (r=0.043) and autonomy (r=0.030), but it was not statistically significant. Only integration of personality (r=0.101, p<0.05), and group oriented attitude (r=0.099, p<0.05) were significantly positively correlated. On the other hand, positive self-evaluation (r= -0.038) and environmental mastery (r= -0.033) were negatively correlated with neuroticism which was not statistically significant.

Extraversion dimension of personality was significantly positively correlated with all the dimensions of mental health viz., positive self-evaluation (r=0.328, p<0.01), perception of reality (r=0.243, p<0.01), integration of personality (r=0.200, p<0.01), autonomy (r=0.290, p<0.01), group oriented attitude (r=0.231, P<0.01), environmental mastery (r=0.231, P<0.01) and overall mental health (r=0.422, P<0.01).

Openness to experience dimension of personality was overall significantly positively correlated with mental health (r=0.306, p<0.01) and all its dimensions i.e., positive self-evaluation (r=0.265, p<0.01), perception of reality (r=0.195, p<0.01), integration of personality (r=0.107, p<0.05), autonomy (r=0.119, p<0.05), group orientation attitude (r=0.270, p<0.01) and environmental mastery (r=0.145, p<0.01).

Agreeableness dimension of personality was positively correlated with mental health ($r=0.075$) and its two dimensions viz., positive self-evaluation ($r=0.045$), and perception of reality ($r=0.000$) but it was not statistically significant. Only integration of personality ($r=0.134$, $p<0.001$), autonomy ($r=0.119$, $p<0.05$) and environmental mastery ($r=0.121$, $p<0.05$) were significantly positive correlated whereas, group oriented attitude dimension of mental health was ($r= -0.129$, $P<0.01$) significantly negatively correlated with agreeableness.

Whereas, Conscientiousness dimension of personality was positively correlated with mental health ($r=0.040$) and all its dimensions viz., positive self-evaluation ($r=0.016$), perception of reality ($r=0.009$), integration of personality ($r=0.076$), autonomy ($r=0.055$) and environmental mastery ($r=0.098$) but group orientation attitude ($r= -0.098$) was negatively correlated and it was not statistically significant.

Table 5: Significance of difference between the mean scores of spiritual intelligence of male and female adolescents (N=400)

Predictor variable	Gender	N	Mean	Std. Deviation	t-value	Sig.
Critical Existence Thinking	Male	200	18.49	4.315	3.30	0.001
	Female	200	16.97	4.84		
Personal Meaning Production	Male	200	15.44	2.55	9.03	0.000
	Female	200	12.92	3.01		
Transcendent Awareness	Male	200	17.66	3.22	7.90	0.000
	Female	200	15.18	3.06		
Conscious State Expansion	Male	200	39.44	5.99	6.74	0.000
	Female	200	35.57	5.46		
Spiritual Intelligence	Male	200	91.02	8.59	11.61	0.000
	Female	200	80.64	9.27		

Table 5 reveals the results of significance of difference of mean and standard deviation of the scores on different dimensions of spiritual intelligence in case of gender. Results show that male adolescents exhibited significantly higher level of critical existence thinking (t=3.30, p<0.001), personal meaning production (t=9.03, p<0.000), transcendental awareness (t=7.90, p<0.000) and conscious state expansion (t=6.74, p<0.000) dimension of spiritual intelligence as compared to female adolescents. Overall male adolescents were significantly higher on spiritual intelligence than female counterparts.

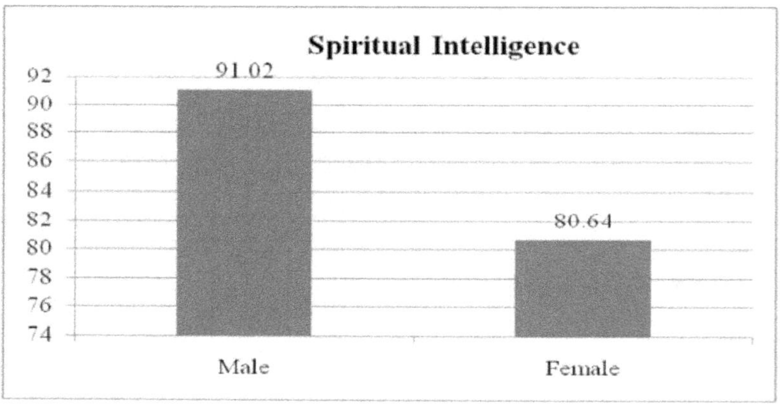

Graphical representation of significance of difference of mean scores of overall spiritual intelligence of male and female adolescents.

Table 6: Significance of difference between the mean scores of resilience of male and female adolescents (N=400)

Predictor	Gender	N	Mean	Std. Deviation	t-value	sig.
Commitment	Male	200	11.50	2.21	4.21	0.000
	Female	200	10.40	2.98		
Problem Solving	Male	200	9.59	1.56	5.06	0.000
	Female	200	8.57	2.41		
Support GMSR	Male	200	9.84	2.06	5.08	0.000
	Female	200	8.68	2.47		
Support HUSR	Male	200	10.89	1.95	7.64	0.000
	Female	200	9.21	2.42		
Role Model	Male	200	3.15	0.93	5.26	0.000
	Female	200	2.60	1.13		
Future Aspirations	Male	200	2.87	0.86	5.01	0.000
	Female	200	2.41	0.99		
Sense of Control	Male	200	5.68	1.46	5.76	0.000
	Female	200	4.74	1.79		
Self-awareness	Male	200	15.92	3.47	2.37	0.018
	Female	200	16.80	3.95		
Resilience	Male	200	69.44	7.53	7.19	0.000
	Female	200	63.40	9.15		

Result Table 6 shows that male adolescents exhibited higher level on commitment ($t=4.21$, $p<0.000$), problem solving ($t=5.06$, $p<0.000$), support GMSR ($t=5.08$, $p<0.000$), support HUSR ($t=7.64$, $p<0.000$), role model ($t=5.26$, $p<0.000$), future aspirations ($t=5.01$, $p<0.000$), and sense of control ($t=5.76$, $p<0.000$) in resilience dimensions as compared to female adolescents. On the other hand, female adolescents exhibited higher on level of self-awareness ($t=2.37$, $p<0.001$) dimension of resilience as compared to male adolescents. Overall male exhibited significantly lower on resilience dimension ($t=7.19$, $p<0.000$) than female adolescents.

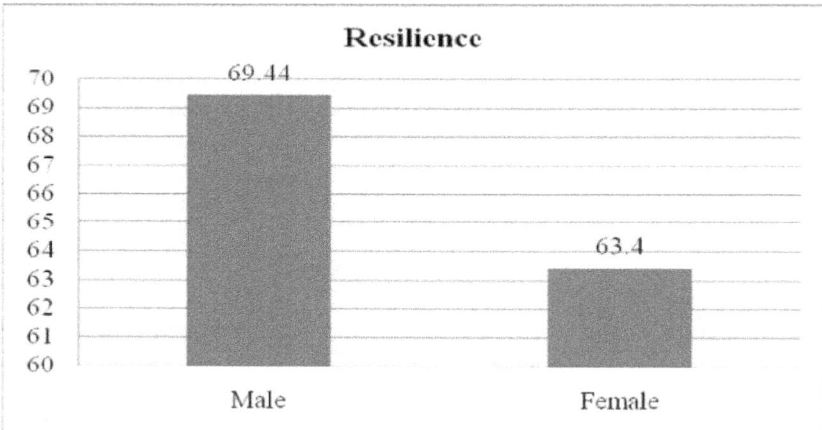

Graphical representation of significance of difference of mean scores of overall resilience of male and female adolescents.

Table 7: Significance of difference between the mean scores of dimensions of personality of male and female adolescents (N=400)

Predictor variable	Gender	N	Mean	Std. Deviation	t-value	sig.
Neuroticism	Male	200	35.74	5.51	-2.99	.003
	Female	200	37.40	5.63		
Extraversion	Male	200	43.49	4.97	10.19	.000
	Female	200	37.40	6.82		
Openness to Experience	Male	200	32.50	4.21	2.87	.004
	Female	200	31.16	5.08		
Agreeableness	Male	200	36.34	6.08	7.89	.000
	Female	200	31.42	6.39		
Conscientiousness	Male	200	40.33	4.88	7.41	.000
	Female	200	36.79	4.66		

Result Table 7 explains that in neuroticism dimension of personality, female adolescents exhibited significantly higher ($t=2.99$, $p<0.003$) than their male counterpart.

In extraversion dimension also male adolescents exhibited significantly higher (t=10.19, p<0.000) as compared to female adolescents. In agreeableness dimension of personality male exhibited significantly higher (t=7.89, p<0.000) as compared to female counterparts. In conscientiousness dimension of personality male exhibited significantly higher (t=7.41, p<0.000) as compared to female adolescents. In openness to experience dimension also male have scored significantly higher (t=2.87, p<0.000) as compared to female adolescents.

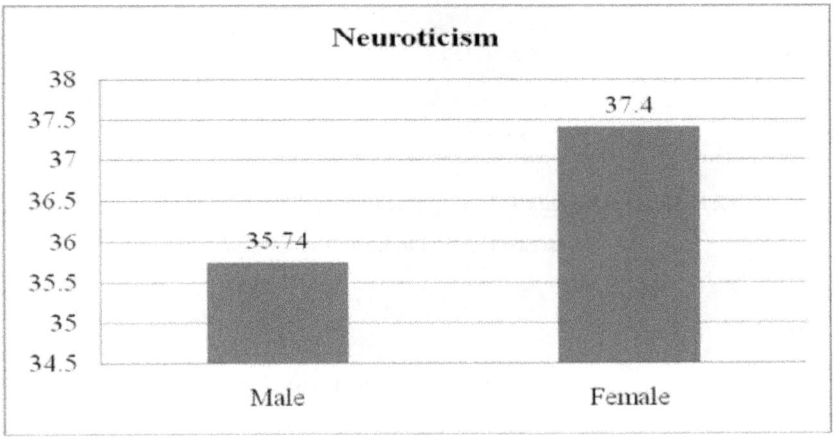

Graphical representation of significance of difference of mean scores of overall neuroticism of male and female adolescents.

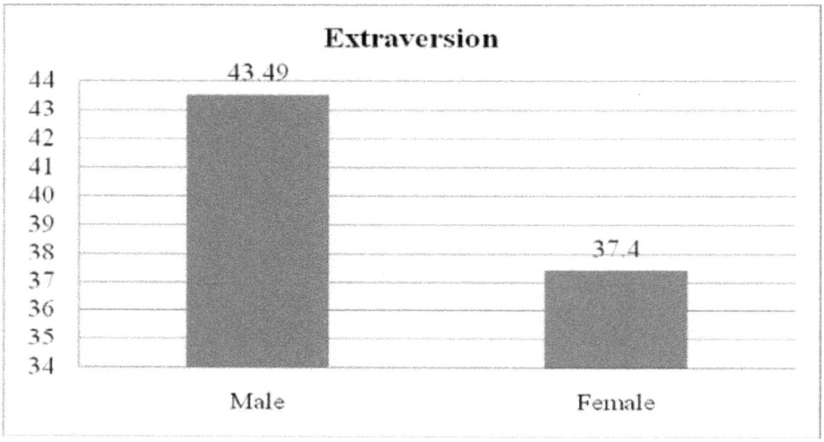

Graphical representation of significance of difference of mean scores of overall extraversion of male and female adolescents.

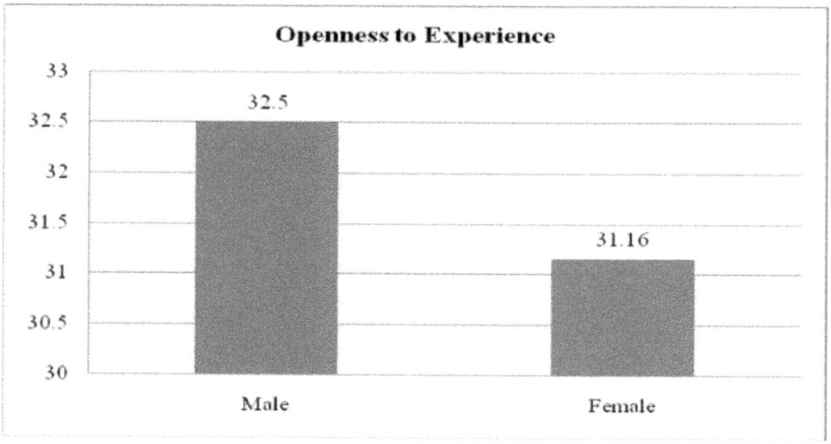

Graphical representation of significance of difference of mean scores of overall openness to experience of male and female adolescents.

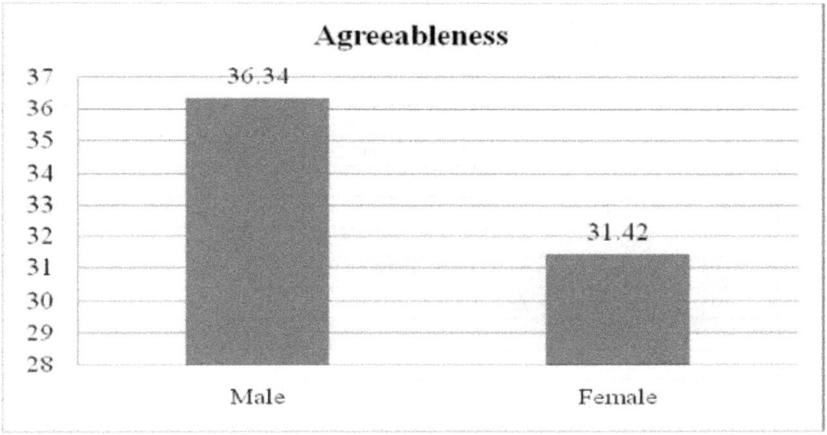

Graphical representation of significance of difference of mean scores of overall agreeableness of male and female adolescents.

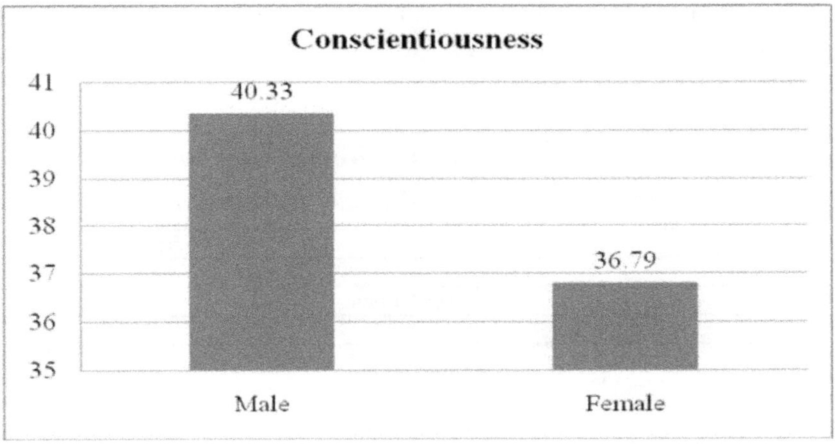

Graphical representation of significance of difference of mean scores of overall conscientiousness of male and female adolescents.

Table 8: Summary of hierarchical regression analysis for personality dimension (neuroticism) as predictor and mental health as criterion

	Mental health	
	Step 1	Step 2
Step I Control Variables		
Age	-0.099	-0.096
Gender	-0.591	-0.614
Family Structure	0.073	0.066
Parent Occupation	-0.021	-0.024
Step 2 predictor variable		(Neuroticism)
β		0.144
R^2	0.363	0.383
ΔR^2	0.363	0.020
ΔF	56.263**	12.960**

**p<0.01, *p<0.05

Table 8 shows the results of hierarchical regression analysis for personality dimension neuroticism as a predictor and overall mental health as a criterion. The results show that after controlling the effect of the demographic variables, neuroticism explains 2.0% of the variance (ΔF=12.960**) in mental health. Above result also indicates that neuroticism is positively related (β = 0.144) to the overall mental health. The standardized regression coefficients (β) are reported in step-1 and step-2.

Table 9: Summary of hierarchical regression analysis for personality dimension (extraversion) as predictor and mental health as criterion

	Mental health	
	Step 1	Step 2
Step I Control Variables		
Age	-0.099	-0.106
Gender	-0.591	-0.500
Family Structure	0.073	0.073
Parent Occupation	-0.021	-0.009
Step 2 predictor variable		Extraversion
β		0.199
R^2	0.357	0.386
ΔR^2	0.368	0.031
ΔF	56.263**	20.213**

**p<0.01, *p<0.05

Table 9 shows the results of hierarchical regression analysis for personality dimension extraversion as a predictor and overall mental health as a criterion. The result shows that after controlling the effect of the demographic variables, extraversion explains 3.1 % of the variance (ΔF= 20.213**) in explaining mental health. Result also indicates that extraversion is positively related (β = 0.199) to overall mental health. The standardized regression coefficients (β) are reported in step-1 and step-2.

Table 10: Summary of hierarchical regression analysis for personality dimension (openness to experience) as predictor and mental health as criterion

	Mental health	
	Step 1	Step 2
Step I Control Variables		
Age	-0.099	-0.090
Gender	-0.591	-0.563
Family Structure	0.073	0.050
Parent Occupation	-0.021	-0.025
Step 2 predictor variable		Openness to experience
β		0.219
R^2	0.357	0.402
ΔR^2	0.363	0.046
ΔF	56.263**	30.913**

**p<0.01, *p<0.05

Table 10 shows the results of hierarchical regression analysis for personality dimension openness to experience as a predictor and mental health as a criterion. The result shows that after controlling the effect of the demographic variables, openness to experience explains 4.6 % of the variance (ΔF=30.913**) in explaining overall mental health. Above result also indicates that openness to experience is positively related to (β = 0.219) overall mental health. The standardized regression coefficients (β) are reported in step-1 and step-2.

Table 11: Summary of hierarchical regression analysis for personality dimension (agreeableness) as predictor and mental health as criterion

	Mental health	
	Step 1	Step 2
Step I Control Variables		
Age	-0.099	-0.091
Gender	-0.591	-0.648
Family Structure	0.073	0.058
Parent Occupation	-0.021	-0.014
Step 2 predictor variable		Agreeableness
β		-0.153
R^2	0.363	0.357
ΔR^2	0.363	0.020
ΔF	56.263**	12.731**

**p<0.01, *p<0.05

Table 11 shows the results of hierarchical regression analysis for agreeableness as a predictor and overall mental health as a criterion. The result shows that after controlling the effect of the demographic variables, agreeableness explains 2.0% (ΔF= 12.731**) in explaining overall mental health. Above result also indicates that agreeableness is negatively related to (β = -0.153) overall mental health. The standardized regression coefficients (β) are reported in step-1 and step-2.

Table 12: Summary of hierarchical regression analysis for personality dimension (Conscientiousness) as predictor and Mental Health as Criterion

	Mental health	
	Step 1	Step 2
Step I Control Variables		
Age	-0.099	-0.076
Gender	-0.591	-0.652
Family Structure	0.073	0.054
Parent Occupation	-0.021	-0.026
Step 2 predictor variable		Conscientiousness
β		-0.172
R^2	0.363	0.380
ΔR^2	0.363	0.025
ΔF	56.263**	16.100**

**p<0.01, *p<0.05

Table 12 shows the result of hierarchical regression analysis for conscientiousness as a predictor and overall mental health as a criterion. The result shows that after controlling the effect of the demographic variables, conscientiousness explains 2.5 % of the variance (ΔF= 16.100**) in explaining overall mental health. Above result also indicates that conscientiousness is negatively related to (β = -0.172) overall mental health. The standardized regression coefficients (β) are reported in step-1 and step-2.

Table 13: Summary of hierarchical stepwise regression analysis for dimension of spiritual intelligence (conscious state expansion, personal meaning production, critical existence thinking, and transcendent awareness) as predictor and mental health as criterion

Model	Variables	Step1	Step 2
Simultaneous Regression	Demographics		
	Age	-0.099	-0.065
	Gender	-0.591	-0.629
	Family Structure	0.073	0.064
	Parent Occupation	-0.099	-0.033
Stepwise Regression	Critical Existence Thinking		0.178
	Personal Meaning Production		-0.169
R		0.602	0.627 0.645
R^2		0.363	0.393 0.416
ΔR^2		0.363	0.030 0.023
ΔF		56.263	19.809 15.451
Sig. F Change		0.000	0.000 0.000

Table 13 shows that after controlling the effect of demographic variables, critical existence thinking and personal meaning production have emerged as a significant predictors to influence the mental health. The result also reveals that on the basis of standardized beta and explained variance critical existence thinking has emerged as the best predictor to influence mental health (β= 0.178) and explain 3.0 % variance in explaining mental health. Personal meaning production emerged as the second-best predictor to influence mental health (β = -0.169) and explains 2.3 % variance in explaining mental health.

Table 14: Summary of hierarchical stepwise regression analysis for dimension resilience (commitment, problem-solving, support GMSR, support HUSR, role model, future aspirations, sense of control, self-awareness) as a predictor and mental health as criterion.

Model	Variables	Step 1	Step 2
Simultaneous Regression	Demographics		
	Age	-0.099	-0.065
	Gender	-0.591	-0.594
	Family Structure	0.073	0.022
	Parent Occupation	-0.021	-0.019
Stepwise Regression	Self-Awareness		-0.261
	Commitment		-0.128
R		0.602	0.653 0.664
R^2		0.363	0.426 0.440
ΔR^2		0.363	0.063 0.015
Δ F		56.263	43.158 10.189
Sig. F Change			0.000 0.002

Table 4 shows that after controlling the effect of demographic variables, self-awareness and commitment have emerged as the significant predictors to influence the mental health. The result also revealed that on the basis of standardized beta self-awareness explains 6.3% variance in explaining mental health and is negatively related to (β= -0.261) mental health, while commitment explains 1.5% variance in explaining mental health and is negatively related (β= -0.128) to mental health.

Table 15: Summary of hierarchical regression analysis for overall spiritual intelligence and overall resilience as predictor and mental health as criterion

	Mental health		
	Step 1	**Step 2**	**Step 3**
Step I Control Variables			
Age	-0.099	-0.100	-0.075
Gender	-0.591	-0.580	-0.683
Family Structure	0.073	0.073	0.047
Parent Occupation	-0.021	-0.022	-0.013
Step 2 predictor variable		spiritual intelligence	
β		0.022	
Step 3 predictor variable Resilience			
β			-0.083
R^2	0.363	0.363	0.433
ΔR^2	0.363	0.000	0.070
ΔF	56.263**	0.229	48.273**

**p<0.01, *p<0.05

Table 15 shows that after controlling the effect of demographic variables, spiritual intelligence does not show the significant influence on mental health. Spiritual intelligence is positively associated (β= 0.022) with mental health. But when resilience is entered in the third step, resilience explains 7.0% variance in explaining mental health and negatively related (β= -0.083) to mental health.

ooo

CHAPTER- V

DISCUSSION

The present research study was mainly undertaken to explain the role of spiritual intelligence, resilience, and personality in the mental health of adolescents. An attempt has been done to analyse and discuss the results recorded in the previous chapter in the light of literature available in the area of investigation. The results are interpreted and discussed accordingly under the following headings.

Relationship between Demographic Variable and Mental Health

Result Table 1 shows the result of correlational analysis revealing that age was negatively correlated with mental health, but it was not statistically significant. Gender was significantly negatively correlated with mental health. Family structure is significantly and positively correlated with mental health. Parent's occupation was not statistically associated with mental health. Demographic variables explain 36.3% variance in mental health which show their significant importance. Family structure and parent occupation is positively correlated with mental health while age and gender is negatively correlated with mental health (females show low mental health as compared to their male counterparts). Previous studies also reported that family structure has been emerged as significant predictor of mental health (Barrett & Turner, 2005; Adlaf and Ivis 1996; Mc Keown et al. 1997). Studies of parent's occupation status like unemployment directly or indirectly predict mental illness (Ihle, Esser, Martin, Blanz, Reis, & Meyer-Probst, 2001). Gender also plays a significant role predicting mental health, gender analysis improves understanding of the epidemiology of mental health problems, decisions, and treatment of these problems in under-reported groups, and also increases the potential for greater public participation in health (Vlassoff, & Garcia Moreno, 2002).

Astbury (2006) found that gender differences in mental disorders extend beyond differences in the rates of various disorders or their differential time of onset or course and include a number of factors that can affect risk or susceptibility, diagnosis, treatment and adjustment to mental disorder. Gender differences in the prevalence of mental disorders vary across age groups. During adolescence, girls have a higher prevalence of depression and eating disorders and engage more in suicidal ideation and suicide attempts than boys. Hawton, Rodham, Evans & Weatherall, (2002), Parker & Roy (2001). In adulthood, women had a higher prevalence of most affective disorders and nonaffective psychosis, and men had higher rates of substance use disorders and antisocial personality disorder, Linzer.et.al (1996).

Relationship between Spiritual Intelligence and Mental Health

In the present study, the first objective was proposed to examine the relationship between spiritual intelligence and mental health of adolescents. It was hypothesized that spiritual intelligence and mental health would be positively correlated. Result Table 2 revealed a significant positive correlation between spiritual intelligence and mental health. The findings are consistent with some of the earliest studies conducted by Lofti and Sayyar (2002) who demonstrated that spiritual intelligence and mental health of adolescents are highly correlated and they also established the concept that there is a considerable relationship between spiritual intelligence and mental health. Similarly Nelms (2005) has also conducted a study on the relationship between spirituality and mental health of college student in a university setting and revealed the positive relationship between the self-reported level of spirituality and the mental health status of college students. Spiritual intelligence is one of the respective types of intelligence that can be developed independently and bring to psychological well-being and overall healthy human development (Perez, 2012). Previous findings on the association between spirituality and mental health have proved that people who consider themselves as spiritually experienced have more potential benefits in terms of low rates of psychological distress, more satisfaction with life and more likely to be high achievers in their goals compared to those who are not spiritual (Corrigan et al., 2003). The role played by spirituality in promoting mental health among different sections of the populations is being widely researched and the findings are impressive with regard to positive associations between the two (Corrigan et al., 2003). Spiritual functions including spiritual intelligence and its components can be used as one of the important instruments to increase individual's mental health (West, 2004).

In a recent study by Pant and Srivastava in the year 2014 on college students revealed that spiritual intelligence and mental health were highly correlated i.e., there is a significant relationship between spiritual intelligence and quality of life and finally, mental health and quality of life. The other study on adolescents' group also reveals that spiritual intelligence and mental health are positively correlated (Singh, 2014).

Others psychologists have also explained a significant positive correlation between spiritual intelligence and nurse's public health (Akbarizadeh, Bagheri, Hatami, & Hajiwandy, 2011).Jain and Purohit (2006) reported the significant differences between spiritual intelligence and mental health ability to use and overcome suffering, ability to transcend pain and being spiritually intelligent about death.

Hosseini et al. (2010) in their adolescence research related to spiritual intelligence and other related theories (Erikson's Theories, 1950; 1968; 1969) discovered that spiritual intelligence had a significant influence on the quality of life and it goes without saying that adolescence is a sensitive period which requires specific training to make a brighter future and exposed from the difficulties. Spirituality can also be viewed as a form of intelligence because it predicts functioning and adaptation and offers capabilities that enable people to solve problems and attain their goals. Yahaya, Momtaz, Othman, Sulaiman & Arisah (2012) have conducted a study to examine the impact of spirituality on adolescents' mental health problems and they found that existential well-being and religious well-being were statistically related with lower odds of mental health problems. Thus, spirituality as a confidence factor might help children to cope with physical and psychological changes through adolescence, fruitfully. In some of the cross-cultural studies it has been presented that western and eastern spirituality in all cultures has positive consequence in growing modification and comfort. Koenig (2012) In the same year, Susana and Ramirez (2012) conducted a longitudinal study in which he showed that spirituality-based coping is associated with increased quality of life and well-being in patients with renal disease and dialysis.

Thus various studies supported the hypothesis of the present study that spiritual intelligence is positively correlated with the mental health of adolescents. Conceiving spirituality as a sort of intelligence extended the psychologists conception of spirituality and allowed its association with the rational cognitive processes like goal achievement and problem solving. Spiritual intelligence is important to construct and develop positive mental health in adolescents.

In this connection Result table 13 has been considered to clarify the results. Spiritual intelligence dimension was further examined as an independent predictor of mental health of adolescents. Hierarchical stepwise regression analysis was applied for the dimensions of spiritual intelligence (conscious state expansion, personal meaning production, critical existence thinking, and transcendent awareness) as a predictor and mental health as a criterion. The obtained result shows that after controlling the influence of the demographic variables, critical existence thinking and personal meaning production have emerged as a significant set of predictors to influence the mental health. The results also revealed that on the basis of standardized beta and explained variance critical existence thinking has emerged as the best predictors to influence mental health and explained 3.0 % variance in prediction of mental health. Personal meaning production emerged as second-best predictor to influence mental health and accounted 2.3 % variance in explaining mental health.

Shabani, Hassan, Ahmad & Baba (2011) reported that mental health can be influenced by spiritual intelligence. Jafar, Hassan, Ahmad and Baba (2011) further examined whether spiritual intelligence can be considered as a predictor for mental health. The result demonstrated that mental health can be influenced by spiritual intelligence. In a study Larson, Sherrill, Lyons, Craigie, Thielman, Greenwold et al. (1992) discovered that 72% of the spiritual obligation variables were advantageous to mental health; input in religious services, social hold up, prayer and rapport with God were favorable in 92% of citations. Consistent with the present result Babanazari et al. (2012) also analyzed the association between spiritual intelligence and contentment for adolescents on a sample of 221 high school students. The outcome of the reading exposed that there was a noteworthy relationship between spiritual intelligence and contentment. Regression investigation showed that consciousness sensing, mystery sensing, value sensing and community sensing considerably projected gladness. In another study Green and Noble (2010) revealed that college and university students are curious to explore the questions regarding spirituality through higher education. An integral approach to the study of consciousness addresses this gap by examining theories of and spirituality from diverse epistemological perspectives, including western science and non-western wisdom traditions. This study explored the intellectual and personal effects of this approach for undergraduate students about consciousness. Results showed that students became more open to diverse ideas about consciousness, more self-aware, and more committed to meditation and self-reflection.

Therefore result supports the hypothesis (H1) that spiritual intelligence would be positively correlated with mental health of adolescents.

Relationship between Resilience and Mental Health

The second objective was proposed to examine the relationship between resilience and mental health of adolescents. It was hypothesized that resilience and mental health would be positively correlated. Result table 3 reveals that resilience is not significantly correlated with mental health. Previous findings show that the individuals who got highest scores in resilience had the lowest levels of depression, anxiety and obsession symptoms (Hjemdal, Vogel, Solem, Hagen and Stiles, 2011). Baldwin et al., (1993) in their study have also reported that non-resilient children had lower mental health scores than resilient children. Pinquart (2009) revealed that individuals with more daily hassles show higher levels of psychological distress and high scores of dispositional resilience were linked to low frequency of stressors, low levels of psychological distress and a decrease in both variables over time. Roy, Sarchiapone, and Carli (2007) found that those who had attempted suicide had significantly lower resilience scores than those who had never attempted suicide. This suggests the possibility that low resilience may be related to poor mental health (depression, in this case). In a study Hartley (2011) examined the relationship between measures of interpersonal resilience, intrapersonal resilience, and mental health with respect to academic and social integration. It was found that there was a strong statistical correlation between the inter-and-intrapersonal (tendency, tolerance of stress and spirituality) resilience factors and mental health.

In another study Besharat (2008) found an inverse correlation between resilience and distress, depression, anxiety and general health problems, and accounted that resilience was positively associated with psychological well-being and negatively associated with psychological distress, depression, and anxiety. Psychological health and vulnerability indices are influenced by different levels of resilience through self-esteem, personal competence and tenacity, tolerance of negative effect, control, and spirituality. Hamid, Keikhosravani, Babamiri, and Dehghani (2012) also reported that there was a positive significant relationship between mental health and resiliency. A very recent study by McGillivray and Pidgeon (2015) on Australian university students examined the attributes of resilient university students, by comparing the differences between high and low resilient students on levels of reported psychological distress, sleep disturbances and mindfulness. Results showed that university students with high levels of resilience reported significantly lower levels of psychological distress and significantly higher levels of mindfulness, compared to university students reporting low levels of resilience.

Some of the Indian studies have been conducted to explain the relationship between resilience and mental health on Indian population. It was done on a group of college-going adolescents. Result showed the positive and inverse both relationship between resiliency and mental health (Kirmani, Sharma, Anas, & Sanam, 2015).

In a very recent study by Hajizadeh, Khalili, Haghighi, & Malekpour, (2016) investigated the role of resiliency and quality of life on the mental health of third-grade high school students. The results showed that resiliency variable has a positive and significant relationship with all components of quality of life (physical health, psychological health, social relationships, and environment). There is a significant relationship between the components of mental health (stress, anxiety and depression) with resiliency and quality of life and its components. Also resilience and quality of life were a significant predictor for the components of mental health (depression, stress, anxiety and depression). This was supported by the study done by Bastaminia, Hashemi, Alizadeh, and Dastoorpoor (2016) observing that there is significant direct (positive) correlation between resilience and all subscales of general health i.e., more the resiliency, the better would be the health conditions.

Thus on the basis of the studies, we can say that with highly resilient adolescents would have better mental health. But these studies do not support the hypothesis of the present study. Resilience is positively correlated with mental health among adolescents. Most of the studies of developmental change have found that increases in individual resilience factors such as self-esteem are age-dependent among children and adolescents. Female adolescents are found to be more likely to report higher levels of communication, empathy, help-seeking, and goals for future and aspirations. They also report more positive connections with parents, teachers and adults in the community, and peers in school and outside school, as well as sense of autonomy experience. These differences, however, show changes over time. The interaction between age and gender is significant for empathy and help-seeking, and for adult support at home, at school and in the community, peer support at school and outside schools, and autonomy experience. (Bolognini *et al*, 1996; Frost & McKelvie, 2004; Watkins *et al*, 1997).

In old age, resilience depends on affective and cognitive reserves and is manifested in coping resources, emotional regulation, motivation, sense of purpose and self-efficacy. One of the assumptions of the lifespan development approach is that resilience tends to increase in old age, rather than decline, acting as a mediator to achieve successful adaptation, otherwise recognized as successful aging (Baltes, 1997).

In this connection has taken as consideration Result table 14 has been considered for more clarification of the results. In result table resilience dimensions were further examined as an independent predictor of mental health of adolescents. Hierarchical stepwise regression analysis was applied for resilience dimension (commitment, problem solving, support GMSR, support HUSR, role model, future aspirations, sense of control, self-awareness) as a predictor and mental health as criterion. The obtained result shows that after controlling the influence of demographic variables, self-awareness and commitment emerged as a significant predictors to influence the mental health. The result also revealed that self-awareness explains 6.3% variance in explaining mental health and is negatively associated with mental health, while commitment explains 1.5% variance in explaining mental health and is negatively associated with mental health. In the other words, we can say that some of the dimensions of resilience significantly predict the mental health among adolescents. In a study Khordzanganeh, Heidarie, and Naderi, (2014) examined the relationship between emotional intelligence, happiness and resiliency with mental health in male and female high school students. The results showed the significant correlation between emotional intelligence, happiness and resiliency with mental health. Also among the predictor variables, resiliency has the stronger ability to predict mental health than happiness and emotional intelligence. Thus the findings add to extend the knowledge about resilience and provide support for schools to develop strategies to promote resilience in students to reduce the risk of developing mental health problems among students. Thus enabling students to flourish under academic pressures may be possible by encouraging their development of the inner strengths of confidence, self-esteem, and responsibility through the building blocks of autonomy and identity.

In Indian context family environment and parenting styles certainly play a very significant role in the psycho-social development of the adolescents. Generally the parents of Indian family always try to fulfill their wishes by pressuring them accordingly. Child feels the academic pressure in his/her home as well. Family socialization experiences may either hinder or enhance the adolescents' ability to cope with the developmental tasks of adolescent as adolescence is the most sensitive period marked by emotional upheavals. Hence, there is a desired need for healthy and supportive family environment to make the adolescents competent, resilient and mentally healthy.

Therefore result does not support the hypothesis (H2) that resilience would be positively correlated with mental health of adolescents.

Relationship between Personality Domains and Mental Health

(1) Relationship between Neuroticism and Mental Health

The third objective was proposed to examine the relationship between personality dimension i.e. neuroticism and mental health of adolescents. It was hypothesized that neuroticism and mental health would be negatively correlated. Result table 4 shows an overall positive correlation between neuroticism dimension of personality and mental health of adolescents, but it was not statistically significant with some of its dimensions are negatively associated with mental health. The past research findings revealed that with the high neuroticism trait, the adolescents would have lower mental health. Zarei, Zeinalipour, Sough, Adli, and Sough (2013) found a negative and significant relationship between neuroticism and general health. In another study Yang, Chiu, Soong, and Chen (2008) explained that neuroticism can be associated with a single episode of a depressive symptom. Shaheen, Jahan, and Shaheen (2014) also reported in their study that there was a significant positive correlation between neuroticism dimension of personality and psychological distress. In a very recent study Mobarakeh, Juhari, Yaacob, Redzuan, and Mobarakeh (2015) also reported that there was a negative relationship between neuroticism trait and adolescent's psychological well-being. According to Costa and McCrae (1992), in a study that people high on neurotic impulsiveness find it difficult to resist temptation or delay gratification while individuals low on conscientious and self-discipline are unable to motivate themselves to perform a task that they would like to accomplish A population varies markedly on neuroticism, ranging from frequent and intense emotional reactions to minor challenges to little emotional reaction even in the face of significant difficulties. Although not widely appreciated, there is growing evidence that neuroticism is a psychological trait of profound public health significance. Neuroticism had the most robust relationship with life satisfaction, suggesting that adolescents who display higher levels of neuroticism are quite likely to experience lower levels of life satisfaction and predictor of many different mental and physical disorders among them. Thus, adolescence may be a crucial time to provide them with adaptive skills (e.g., emotion regulation, coping strategies, and interpersonal skills) while they are open to exploring and discovering their personal identities.

Family plays an important role in adolescents' personal, social and academic achievement. Although socialization and life experiences modify personality traits and influence how they have been exposed. In today's contexts we can see that in our Indian society are giving equal rights to girls and boys and adolescents experiencing supportive environment from their family, school and society. This could be one of the possible explanations.

Therefore results do not support the hypothesis (H3) (a) that neuroticism would be negatively correlated with mental health of adolescents

(2) Relationship between Extraversion and Mental Health

The third objective was proposed to examine the relationship between personality domain i.e. extraversion and mental health of adolescents. It was hypothesized that extraversion dimension of personality and mental health of adolescents would be positively correlated. Result table 4 indicates that with the high score on extraversion domain of personality the adolescents would have better mental health. The results are also consistent with some of the earlier findings. Zarei, Zeinalipour, Sough, Adli, and Sough (2013) found a positive and significant relationship between personality traits of extraversion and general health. In another study Shaheen, Jahan and Shaheen (2014) reports that extraversion domain was negatively correlated with psychological distress and positive correlation with psychological well-being (Mobarakeh, Juhari, Yaacob, Redzuan and Mobarakeh, 2015). On the basis of present findings we can say that extraverted individuals reported better mental health and higher quality of life. The reasons could be that liking people and prefer large group and gatherings, extraverts are also assertive, active and talkative. They like excitement and stimulation and tend to be cheerful in disposition. They are upbeat, energetic, and optimist in any environmental situation. Extraversion is the act, state, or habit of being predominantly concerned with and obtaining gratification from what is outside the self, defined as "a trait characterized by a keen interest in other people and external events, and venturing forth with confidence into the unknown (Ewen, 1998).The broad dimension of extraversion encompasses such more specific traits as talkative, energetic, gregarious and assertiveness.

Therefore results supported the hypothesis H3 (b) that there would be positive correlation between extraversion and mental health.

(3) Relationship between Openness to Experience and Mental Health

The third objective was proposed to examine the relationship of personality domain i.e. openness to experience and mental health of adolescents. It was hypothesized that openness to experience and mental health of adolescents would be positively correlated. Result table 4 indicates a significant positive correlation between openness to experiences domain of personality and mental health of adolescents, which means that with high in openness to experience domain of personality adolescents would have better mental health. The findings are consistent with some of the earliest studies. For example, Zarei, Zeinalipour, Sough, Adli, and Sough (2013) found a positive and significant relationship between personality traits of openness (flexibility) and general health. Researches have also explained that there is a significant relationship between openness to experience and mental health (Haren et al., 2003). In a recent study Shirazi, Khan and Ansari (2002) & Sadeghi, Ofoghi and Azizi (2015) examined the relationship between mental health and openness to experience of students and revealed the same result that there was a positive relationship between openness to experience with mental health. Thus, it is necessary that adolescents should be equipped with appropriate abilities, skills, and knowledge so that they can have a better adjustment with their society at large. It includes traits like having wide interests, being imaginative, insightful, attentiveness to inner feelings, preference for variety, and intellectual curiosity (Costa, & McCrae, 1992)

Therefore results supported the hypothesis H3 (c) that openness to experiences and mental health would be positively correlated.

(4) Relationship between Agreeableness and Mental Health

The third objective was proposed to examine the relationship of personality domain i.e. agreeableness and mental health of adolescents. It was hypothesized that agreeableness and mental health of adolescents would be positively correlated. Result table 4 indicates a positive correlation between agreeableness and mental health of adolescents, which means that with the high score on agreeableness domain of personality, adolescents would have better mental health. The result is consistent with some of the earliest studies. In a study Zarei, Zeinalipour, Sough, Adli, and Sough, (2013) revealed a positive and significant relationship between personality traits of agreeableness and general health. It was corroborated with the findings of Mobarakeh,

Juhari, Yaacob, Redzuan, and Mobarakeh (2015) & Cheng, Weiss and Siegel (2015) stating that agreeableness traits would have a positive correlation with psychological well-being. This type of person is sympathetic to other and eager to help them and believes that other will be equally helpful in return. These domains describe personality both as socially preferable as well as psychologically healthier. Agreeableness measures how compatible the person is with other people, or basically how able he/she is to get along with others. It is a tendency to be pleasant and accommodating in social situations reflecting individual differences in concern for cooperation and social harmony (Graziano & Eisenberg 1997). Agreeable traits include empathetic, considerate, friendly, generous, and helpful and they also have an optimistic view of human nature. They tend to believe that most people are honest, decent, and trustworthy and less likely to suffer from social rejection (Bierman, 2003).

Therefore results the proposed hypothesis H3 (d) that agreeableness and mental health would be positively correlated.

(5) Relationship between Conscientiousness and Mental Health

The third objective was proposed to examine the relationship of personality domain i.e. conscientiousness and mental health of adolescents. It was hypothesized that conscientiousness and mental health of adolescents would be positively correlated. Result table 4 indicates a positive correlation between conscientiousness and mental health of adolescents, which means that with the high scores of conscientiousness domain of personality, adolescents would have better mental health. The findings are consistent with some of the earliest studies i.e., Zarei, Zeinalipour, Sough, Adli, and Sough (2013) again explored a positive and significant relationship between personality traits of conscientiousness and general health. Shaheen, Shaheen, and Shaheen (2013) also revealed that conscientiousness dimension of personality has a significant and positive relation better mental health among students. In an extensive review of the study reported that conscientiousness-related traits were negatively related to all risky health-related behaviors and positively related to all beneficial health-related behaviors (Bogg & Roberts, 2004). It is now well-established that conscientiousness predicts health and longevity in various populations and over long periods of time (Kern & Friedman, 2008; Roberts et al., 2007). Conscientious adolescents usually grow up to smoke less, eat healthier foods, wear seat belts, and engage in a range of other healthy behaviors (Bogg & Roberts, 2004; Lodi-Smith et al., 2010). Self-control is an active process of planning, organizing and carrying out the task and individual differences in this tendency are the basis of conscientiousness. The Conscientious individual is purposeful strong-willed and determined and have better mental health. People with conscientiousness personalities were found to be organized thoroughly. They plan ahead and also related to impulse control, but it should not be confused with the problems of impulse control found in neuroticism

Therefore results supported the hypothesis H3 (e) that conscientiousness and mental health would be positively correlated.

The fifth objective was proposed to verify the contribution of spiritual intelligence, resilience, and personality in the prediction of mental health of adolescents and relative importance of these variables. It was hypothesized that spiritual intelligence, resilience, and personality would significantly predict the mental health of adolescents. Considering Table (8-12) it was further examined through the hierarchical regression for mental health as criterion and personality dimension as a predictor. The findings of the present study also advanced the knowledge about the various personality factors which are the indicators of mental health among adolescents. The findings revealed that after controlling the effect of the demographic variables, the personality trait neuroticism explains 2.0% of the variance, extraversion explains 3.1% of the variance, openness to experience explains 4.6% of the variance, agreeableness explains 2.0% of the variance, and conscientiousness explains 2.5% of explaining the variance in overall mental health. However, the magnitude of their contribution was relatively small but the contributions of the personality domain were statistically significant. In this connection, Shirazi and Khan (2012) examined the relationship between mental health and personality characteristics among students. The result shows that there is a significant correlation between mental health and personality characteristics. The multiple regression analysis using the stepwise method found agreeableness, neuroticism, and openness as significant predictors of mental health. Early detection for indications of mental health problems and understanding factors contributing to stress among students would promote a better understanding of mental health in future and findings suggest that more researches are required to know about students' mental health and personality characteristics at length.

The finding corroborated with previous finding. In a very recent study Cheng, Weiss, & Siegel (2015) also examined the relative contributions of individual characteristics of personality and health behaviors to subjective well-being among university-attending emerging young adults. Three dimensions of well-being were assessed viz., effective (positive affect), physical/mental (overall health), and cognitive (quality of life). Extraverted individuals reported more positive affect and higher quality of life. Neuroticism was associated with the less positive effect, poorer health, and lower quality of life. Physical activity was consistently associated with subjective well-being, accounting for 33%, 13%, and 32% of the total variance in a positive affect, overall health and quality of life respectively. Findings indicate that health behaviors are important correlates of three dimensions of well-being over and above the effects of personality traits.

Overall findings of present study revealed that different personality factors play an important role with mental health. Agreeableness, openness, extraversion, and conscientiousness are positively correlated with mental health. In other words adolescents with this type of personality would certainly display better mental health. Whereas neuroticism was negatively associated with mental health of adolescents, it means that the adolescents with neurotic personality would have a lower level of mental health. All personality dimensions significantly predict the mental health of adolescents.

Hence results support the hypothesis H5 that spiritual intelligence, resilience, and personality would significantly predict the mental health of adolescents.

Prediction of Hierarchical Regression Analyses for Overall Spiritual Intelligence and Overall Resilience as Predictor and Mental Health as Criterion.

Result table 15 shows that after controlling the influence of demographic variables, spiritual intelligence does not show the significant influence on mental health. Spiritual intelligence is positively correlated (β= 0.022) to mental health. In third step, resilience is entered and it explains 7.0% variance in mental health and negatively associated (β= -0.083) with mental health. In a study regarding resilience spiritual intelligence and mental health. Hamid, Keikhosravani, Babamiri, and Dehghani (2012) investigated the relationship between mental health, spiritual intelligence and resiliency among the Kermanshah Medical Science University. The results indicated that there was a positive significant relationship between mental health and resiliency. Also, there was a positive significant relationship between spiritual intelligence and resiliency. The results of multiple regressions showed that the mental health had played an important role to predict resiliency. They concluded that mental health and spiritual intelligence had a significant role to predict resiliency. Where people with a higher degree of mental health would have higher degrees of resiliency to increase mental health, and spiritual intelligence can rebound to increase of resiliency.

In a very recent study by Hajizadeh, Khalili, Haghighi, & Malekpour in year 2016 investigated the role of resiliency and quality of life on mental health of third grade high school students and reported that resilience and quality of life were a significant predictors for explaining the components of mental health (depression, stress, and anxiety). In another study, Ebrahimi Dehghani & others (2012) indicated that there was a positively meaningful relationship between resiliency and mental health, and also the spiritual intelligence and resiliency. Results of multiple regressions analysis indicated that mental health and spiritual intelligence meaningfully explain resiliency. Mental health has a more significant role in predicting and explaining resiliency.

Comparison of spiritual Intelligence of adolescents with respect to gender

The fourth objective was proposed to examine the gender difference in spiritual intelligence. It was hypothesized that spiritual intelligence would be higher in boys as compared to girls. Result table 5 and figure 1explains that males have scored better on spiritual intelligence scores than female adolescents. The result contradicts with some of the earliest studies. For example in a study, Jeloudar et.al (2010) and Kushwaha (2012) reported that the female has higher level of spiritual intelligence as compared to their male counterpart. Similarly, Singh (2011) revealed that girls had significantly higher level of spiritual intelligence as compared to boys. Similarly, Khan and Singh, (2013) indicated significant gender differences among male and female teachers on spirituality i.e., females were found higher on spiritual intelligence than males. Again Nangia, (2014) revealed that female students had higher spiritual intelligence as compared to male students. Whereas in some studies it was reported that male student was superior in spiritual intelligence as compared to female (Gupta, 2012; Nazam, 2014).

However, maximum number of recent studies show mixed finding regarding in terms of spiritual intelligence (Siddiqui, 2013; Kaur, & Singh, 2013; Jafari et al., 2014). In a very recent study by Kotnala, (2015) revealed that there is no significant difference between male and female students on conscious state expansion, critical existential thinking, personal meaning production and transcendental awareness dimension of spiritual intelligence. In another study Kushwaha, (2014) reported that there is no significant difference between the spiritual intelligence of male and female prospective teachers. This study also reveals that male prospective teachers have the same level in inner-self, inter-self, biostoria, life perspectives, spiritual actualization and value orientation as compared to their counterpart's. Present study is based on those adolescents who are studying in his schools. Education is an important tool which plays a crucial role to overcome the gender differences in society. So it may be a reason that no gender difference was found in some study.

Therefore result supported the hypothesis H4 (a) spiritual intelligence would be higher in boys as compared to girls.

Comparisons of resilience of adolescents with respect to gender

The fourth objective was proposed to examine the gender differences in resilience. It was hypothesized that resilience would be higher in boys as compared to girls. Result table 6 reveals a significant gender differences on resilience scores. The results are consistent with some of the earliest studies. In a study Kamble (2015) Shanahan and Hofer (2005); and Al-Naser and Sandman (2000) reports significant gender differences on resilience and finding are also supported by the studies (Campbell-Sills et al., 2009; von Soest et al., 2010; Waktaar and Torgersen, 2012; Abukari and Laser, 2013; Stratta et al., 2013; Ying et al., 2014) stating higher resilience in adolescents male as compared to female. Among older populations, males have also been reported higher on resilience as compared to female (Boardman et al., 2008). In a study Yu and Zhang (2007) demonstrated that in chinese community men were more resilient than women. But some of the earlier studies show contradictory findings stating that female has high resiliency than males. Somchit and Sriyaporn's (2004) studied resilience on adolescent group, Banyard and Cantor's (2004) investigation on college students, and Sun and Stewart's (2007) investigation on children reported that females showed greater resilience than males.

As far as Indian study is concerned Kaur and Kaur (2012) also reported that female adolescents found to be more resilient than male adolescents. Some of the other empirical literature indicates that females have higher resilience than males in diverse groups such as children (Werner, 1985; Sun and Stewart, 2007; Riches et al., 2009), adolescents (Chung and Elias, 1996; Hair et al., 2001; Hampel and Petermann, 2005; Arokiaraj et al., 2011) and adults (Netuveli et al., 2008; Wagnield, 2011; Ma et al., 2013). Investigating academic resilience and gender in higher education in African

American and Hispanic participants, it was found that females faced greater resistance than males in the pursuit of their career goals (Morales', 2008). Grotberg (1997) agrees that despite perceiving more adversity than males, females are found to use resilience factors such as trusting relationships and finding support more than males. On the other hand, some studies reported that there is no significant difference between male and female students on resiliency (Ebrahimi Dehghani & others, 2012; Chukwuoji & Ajaero, 2014; Sreehari & Nair (2015).

Resilience is not a function of gender (Collishaw et al., 2007), and Jaffee, Caspi, Moffitt, Polo-Tomas and Taylor (2007) posited that males and females were equally likely to be resilient. Individual strengths played a more important role in distinguishing resilient from non-resilient males and females. In this study, the dimension of the resilience scale has focused on social competence, problem-solving skills, autonomy and sense of purpose. Considering the socio-cultural environment here, it may be noted that these attributes are more encouraged in males than females, by both societies as well as in females themselves.

Therefore results supported the hypothesis H4 (b) that resilience would be higher in boys as compared to girls.

Comparison of neuroticism dimension of personality of adolescents with respect to gender

The fourth objective was proposed to examine the gender difference in one of the dimension of personality i.e. neuroticism. It was hypothesized that neuroticism would be higher in girls as compared to boys. The result table 7 and figure 3 reveals significant gender differences on neuroticism dimension of personality among adolescents. The results are consistent with some of the earliest studies. Goodwin and Gotlib (2004), Vianello, Schnabel, Sriran, and Nosek (2013) Shaheen, Jahan and Shaheen (2014) and Weisberg, DeYoung, and Hirsh (2011) reports the higher levels of neuroticism among females than males. In another study Chapman, Duberstein, Sörensen, and Lyness (2008) revealed higher levels of neuroticism in older women than older men. However, some studies reported no gender differences on the dimension of neuroticism (Branje et al., 2007). In a recent by Study Sharma and Gulati in 2015 also reported neuroticism was nearly equal in both males and females.

Female adolescents generally experience negative emotional states and such feelings such as anxiety, anger, guilt, and depressed mood found so that they respond more poorly to environmental stress, are more likely to interpret ordinary situations as threatening and minor frustrations as hopelessness more difficult. They are often self-conscious and shy, and they may have trouble controlling urges and delaying gratification. Neuroticism is associated with low emotional intelligence, which involves emotional regulation, motivation, and interpersonal skills. It is also a risk factor for "internalizing" mental disorders such as phobia, depression, panic disorder, and other anxiety disorders traditionally called neuroses (Hettema, Neale, Myers, Prescott, & Kendler 2006). Individuals who are high in neuroticism may show more emotional reactions whenever confronted with stressful situations (Van Heck, 1997). Moreover, they seem to use avoiding and distracting coping strategies, such as denying, wishful thinking, and self-criticism, rather than more approaching strategies (Bolger, 1990; Heppner et al., 1995; McCrae & Costa, 1986). This could be the possible reason that females are more neurotic as compared to males.

Therefore results supported the hypothesis H4 (c) that neuroticism would be higher in girls as compared to boys.

Comparison of extraversion dimension of personality of adolescents with respect to gender

The fourth objective was proposed to examine the gender difference in dimension of personality i.e. extraversion. It was hypothesized that extraversion would be higher in boys as compared to girls. Result table 7 reveal a significant gender differences on extraversion dimension of personality among adolescents. The result corroborates with some of the earliest studies. Branje, Van Lieshout, and Gerris (2007) reported that boys tended to be more extroverted than girls. Whereas in some findings it has been reported that females were more extroverted than males (Costa, McCrae, & Martin, 2008). Same result described by McCrae, Costa, et al., (2005), McCrae et al., (2002), Weisberg, DeYoung and Hirsh (2011), and Goodwin and Gotlib (2004). Sharma, and Gulati (2015), Shaheen, Jahan and Shaheen (2014) and Vianello, Schnabel, Sriran, and Nosek (2013) also reported that females scored higher on extraversion dimension of personality than among males. Extraversion is the act, state, or habit of being predominantly concerned with and obtaining gratification from what is outside the self, and venturing forth with confidence into the unknown (Ewen, 1998).The broad dimension of extraversion encompasses more specific traits as talkative, energetic, gregarious and assertiveness.

Therefore the results supported the hypothesis H4 (d) that boys would score higher on extraversion as compared to girls.

Comparison of openness to experience dimension of personality of adolescents with respect to gender

The fourth objective was proposed to examine the gender difference in dimension of personality i.e. openness to experience. It was hypothesized that openness to experience would be higher in boys as compared to girls. Result table 7 and figure 7 reveal a significant gender differences on openness to experience dimension of personality among adolescents. The result is consistent with some of the earliest studies. In a study Branje, Van Lieshout, and Gerris (2007) reported that boys tended to be more open to experience than girls. In another study, Goodwin and Gotlib (2004) revealed that level of openness to experience dimension was significantly higher among males as compared to females. Vianello, Schnabel, Sriran, and Nosek (2013) observed a higher level of openness to experience in men than women. Similarly, Shaheen, Jahan, and Shaheen (2014) also reported in a study that male had significantly higher level of openness to experiences than female. Women reported themselves to be higher in openness to feelings whereas men were higher in openness to ideas (Costa, Terracciano & Mc Crae, 2001). Openness is the most significant predictor of psychometric intelligence (e.g., Heaven & Ciarrochi, 2012). It is also associated with the acquisition of knowledge composing crystallized intelligence, such as information and vocabulary (Bates & Rock, 2004). In Indian context male adolescents with high scores in openness dimention are more motivated to participate in different kinds of intellectual activities from reading literature to visiting museums exhibitions and extra co curricular activities. These are the plausible reasons that boys are rich in openness to experience dimension of personality as compared to girls.

Therefore result support the hypothesis H4 (e) that boys would score higher on openness to experience as compared to girls.

Comparisons of agreeableness dimension of personality of adolescents with respect to gender

The fourth objective was proposed to examine the gender difference in dimension of personality i.e. agreeableness. It was hypothesized that agreeableness would be higher in boys as compared to girls. Result table 7 and figure 5 reveal a significant gender differences on agreeableness dimension of personality among adolescents. The findings are consistent with earlier studies. In a recent study Shaheen, Jahan and Shaheen (2014) found that male adolescents scored significantly higher on agreeableness as compared to female counterparts. However, most of studies show that female had high level of agreeableness as compared to male adolescents (Feingold, 1994; Costa, Terracciano, & McCrae, 2001; Goodwin & Gotlib, 2004; Chapman, Duberstein, Sörensen, and Lyness 2008; Weisberg, DeYoung & Hirsh, 2011; Vianello, Schnabel, Sriran, Nosek, 2013). The other previous studies, also reported no gender difference. Branje et al. (2007) found no gender differences on agreeableness dimensions of personality. Indian male adolescents are compatible with other people, or basically how able they are to get along with others. It is a tendency to be pleasant and accommodating in social situations reflecting individual differences in concern for cooperation and social harmony (Graziano & Eisenberg 1997). Agreeable traits include empathetic, considerate, friendly, generous, and helpful and they also have an optimistic view of human nature. They tend to believe that most people are honest, decent, and trustworthy and less likely to suffer from social rejection (Bierman, 2003). In addition, evidence have shown that whereas most people are likely to help their own kin, or empathies with them but contrarily, agreeable people are likely to help even when these conditions are not present (Graziano, Habashi, Sheese, & Tobin 2007) thus being traited for helping and do not need any other motivation (Penner, Fritzsche, Craiger, & Freifeld, 1995).

Therefore the results support the proposed hypothesis H4 (d) that boys would score higher on agreeableness as compared to girls.

Comparison of conscientiousness dimension of personality of adolescents with respect to gender

The fourth objective was proposed to examine the gender difference in dimension of personality i.e. conscientiousness. It was hypothesized that conscientiousness would be higher in boys as compared to girls. Result table 7 reveals a significant gender differences on conscientiousness dimension of personality among adolescents. The result is also consistent with some of the earliest studies. Shaheen, Jahan, and Shaheen (2014) found that male students scored significantly higher on conscientiousness as compared to female students. However, Vianello, Schnabel, Sriran, and Nosek (2013) examined gender differences in implict and explict personality traits, in which they reported gender differences in conscientiousness. However, very recently Raut and Mundada (2016) reports in their study that boys and girls do not significantly differ in the dimension of conscientiousness, but means scores shows that boys had higher scores than girls. The results also show that there is a significant difference between the anxiety of boys and girls students. Female are more anxious than male adolescents because the female adolescents are generally economically dependent on their parents and they are more oriented towards family work and responsibility. Though the scenario is constantly changing. These factors include ever increasing competition, adjustment with day to day life, family adaptation, and the field chosen for education, their aim, etc. Conscientiousness is one of the best predictors of performance in the workplace and conscientious adolescents are generally more reliable, more motivated and hard working. Female nurturing behaviors depend upon socialization of feminine gender role and male have significantly higher thrill and adventure seeking than female.

Therefore results support the proposed hypothesis H4 (d) that boys would score higher on conscientiousness as compared to girls.

Overall findings suggest that demographic variables explain maximum variance in mental health than others variable like spiritual intelligence, resilience, and personality which shows their significant importance. After controlling the demographic variable resilience has been emerged as the best predictor to influence the mental health as compared to spiritual intelligence and other personality factors.

CHAPTER- VI

SUMMARY AND CONCLUSIONS

Adolescents go through many changes and challenges in a short period of time. Adolescence as a formative stage plays a significant role in the study of developmental psychopathology because after this maturational interval it is difficult to change some behavioural and emotional patterns. Thus, this period is a very important period of life as it lays the foundation for the future of an individual.

Resilience is the phenomenon of achieving favourable outcomes despites adversity. In other words, the identification of resilience is based on two fundamental judgments first, it involves exposure to a significant challenge and second it refers to competence achieved under such adversity. Resilience is understood to play an important role in helping an individual navigate through the major transitional point in life. The present study has expanded the literature by providing corroborating support from previous researches that has identified links between spiritual intelligence, resilience, personality and mental health of adolescents.

The study unveils that there is a significant gender difference in spiritual intelligence, resilience, personality and mental health of adolescents. The study also reveals that spiritual intelligence, resilience and mental health are significantly positively correlated, whereas personality factors viz., openness, conscientiousness, extraversion, and agreeableness are positively correlated with mental health and neuroticism is negatively correlated with mental health. Furthermore, this study also identifies that resilience emerged as the best predictor of mental health in adolescents. So enhancing the spiritual intelligence may result in better outcomes in mental health as it in the study. Personality factors also influence the mental health of adolescents. Thus, we conclude that resilience, spiritual intelligence, and personality factors are relevant for maintaining the sound mental health of adolescents.

Thus the purpose of the present study was to examine the role of spiritual intelligence, resilience, and personality in mental health of adolescents.

Objectives

The study was conducted to test the following major objectives:

1. To examine the relationship between spiritual intelligence and mental health of adolescents.
2. To examine the relationship between resilience and mental health of adolescents.
3. To examine the relationship between personality and mental health of adolescents.
4. To examine the gender differences in spiritual intelligence, resilience, and personality.
5. To verify the contribution of spiritual Intelligence, resilience, and personality in the prediction of mental health of adolescents and relative importance of these variables.

Hypotheses

Based on prior finding and theoretical background the following hypotheses were framed on the basis of research objectives.

H1: Spiritual intelligence would be positively correlated with mental health of adolescents.

H2: Resilience would be positively correlated with mental health of adolescents.

H3 (a): Neuroticism dimension of personality would be negatively correlated with mental health of adolescents.

(b): Extraversion dimension of personality would be positively correlated with mental health of adolescents.

(c): Openness to experience dimension of personality would be positively correlated with mental health of adolescents (d): Agreeableness dimension of personality would be positively correlated with mental health of adolescents.

(e): Conscientiousness dimension of personality would be positively correlated with mental health of adolescents.

H4 (a): Spiritual intelligence would be higher in boys as compared to girls.

(b): Resilience would be higher in boys as compared to girls.

(c): Girls would score higher on neuroticism as compared to boys.

(d): Boys would score higher on extraversion, agreeableness, and conscientiousness as compared to girls.

(e): Boys would score higher on openness to experience as compared to girls.

H5: Spiritual intelligence, resilience, and personality would significantly predict the mental health of adolescents.

Methodology

Design

In the present study, an attempt has been made to examine the relationship of spiritual intelligence, resilience, personality and mental health of adolescents. The present study follows a correlational design. Spiritual intelligence, resilience and personality have been treated as predictors and mental health as criterion variable among adolescents. Hence in order to obtained detailed information from a relatively large number of cases, the most suitable method i.e. simple descriptive survey was used.

Sample

The present research study was conducted on a sample of 400 students (200 male and 200 female) aged 17 to 19 years. The students were selected from different schools of Varanasi city.

Measures

The following measures were employed to verify the proposed hypotheses.

1. Personal Data Blank
2. Mental Health Inventory
3. Resilience Scale
4. Personality Inventory (NEO-FFI)
5. King's Spiritual intelligence scale

1. **Personal Data Blank-** In order to obtain relevant personal information about the respondent included in the sample, a personal data sheet (Hindi) was designed by the researcher. Information related to name, age, gender, caste, sex, residential background, address, birth order, and type of family etc were included in the sheet. They were instructed to fill this sheet before the completion of all four standardized tests.

2. **Mental Health Inventory (M.H.I)** – Mental Health Inventory (M.H.I.) developed by Jagdish & A.K. Srivastava (1996) was used for measuring mental health of individuals in various sphere of life and has been designed to measure mental health (positive) of normal individuals. The Mental Health Inventory consists of 56 items and six popular indices i.e. positive self-evaluation (PSE), perception of reality (PR), integration of personality (IP), autonomy (AUTNY), group-oriented attitudes (GOA), and environmental mastery (EM). The alpha values of these indices are 0.75, 0.71, 0.72, 0.72, 0.74, 0.71 and 0.73 respectively.
3. **Resilience Scale-** Resilience Scale originally developed by Mampane (2005) was used for the purpose of identifying resilient and non-resilient adolescents. The scale consists of 25 items based on the following resilience factors i.e., Commitment, future aspirations, problem-solving, role models, self-awareness, sense of control and support. The statements are short, simple and easy to understand and reflect descriptions of behaviors that relate to activities, events and characteristics assumed relevant and applicable to an adolescent's life. The reliability of this scale was established at an alpha value 0.82.

4. **NEO-FFI-** Personality traits of adolescents was measured by the NEO Five- Factor Inventory (NEO-FFI), which was originally developed by Costa and Mc Care in 1992. The NEO-FFI is a well recognized, extensively tested and widely used scale to measure the Big Five Personality dimensions (e.g. Mooradian & Olver, 1997; Renner, 2002). This inventory consists of sixty items (twelve items for each factor) and based on five-point Likert format (from "strongly agree" to "strongly disagree").

   Reliability (Cronbach's Alpha) is 0.85 for neuroticism, 0.80 for extraversion, 0.75 for agreeableness, 0.83 for conscientiousness factor and 0.66 for openness.

5. **King's Spiritual intelligence scale:** The spiritual intelligence self-report questionnaire developed by King (2008) was used for measurement of spiritual intelligence. This Spiritual intelligence scale consists of 24 items and four indices i.e. existential thinking, transcendental awareness, personal meaning production, and conscious state expansion. The Cronbach's alpha coefficient is 0.95 and the obtained reliability from bisections is 0.84.

   Hindi adaptation of all questionnaires was done by the researcher during the course of study.

Analyses and results

The obtained data were statistically analyzed in term of mean, standard deviation, t-test, the coefficient of correlation, hierarchical regression analyses and hierarchical stepwise regression analyses.

Major Findings

Major findings of the study are given below:

1. Demographic variables explain 36.3% variance in mental health which shows their significance. Family structure and parental occupation are positively associated with mental health while age and gender are negatively associated with mental health (females show low mental health as compared to their male counterparts).

2. Results of correlational analysis for spiritual intelligence and all its dimensions with mental health show that spiritual intelligence and its dimensions are positively and significantly associated with mental health, only conscious state expansion is significantly negatively associated with mental health. Hierarchical regression of dimension of the spiritual intelligence shows that self-awareness and commitment have emerged as significant predictors to influence the mental health of adolescents.
3. On the basis of correlational analysis overall resilience is negatively associated with mental health. Hierarchical regression of dimension of resilience shows that self-awareness and commitment emerged as a significant predictor to influence the mental health of adolescents.
4. The coefficient of correlation was computed to examine the relationship between personality dimension and mental health. Result revealed that extraversion, agreeableness, conscientiousness, and openness to experience is positively and significantly correlated with the mental health of adolescents. The results of correlational analyses between neuroticism and mental health show that neuroticism is negatively associated with mental health of adolescents. Hierarchical regression of dimension of personality shows that all personality traits i.e., neuroticism extraversion, openness to experience, agreeableness, and conscientiousness have emerged as significant predictors. Though the magnitude of their contribution was relatively small but the contributions of the personality dimensions were statistically significant.
5. The results of the significance of difference(t-test) between male and female adolescents on spiritual intelligence and all its dimensions show that male adolescents have scored higher on spiritual intelligence and all its dimensions as compared to female adolescents and this difference(t-test) between male and female adolescents on resilience and all its dimensions shows that male adolescents have scored higher on resilience as compared to female adolescents and this difference was found significant.
6. The findings of the study also unveils that male adolescents have scored higher on agreeableness, conscientiousness, openness, and extraversion as

compared to their female counterparts. The findings also revealed that female adolescents scored higher on neuroticism as compared to male adolescents.

7. Overall findings suggest that resilience is significantly and positively associated with mental health. Resilience has emerged as the best predictor to influence the mental health as compared to spiritual intelligence, and personality.

Implications

- The most important implication of the study is that it opens a new horizon in front of school teachers and also the parents of the adolescent to realize the importance of paying attention to the spirituality in the growth of mental health of adolescents as spiritual intelligence is necessary for discernment in making spiritual choices that contribute to psychological well-being and overall healthy human development.
- Another important implication of the study is to give a new insight to adolescents in order to develop the concept of spiritual intelligence in their daily life. Spiritual intelligence helps people to reduce their negative emotions and benefit from appropriate strategies to manage stress and solve life problems to minimize anxiety.
- When spiritual intelligence is high, the person (individual) appears to be more intellectual. On the other hand, when spiritual intelligence is low, individuals show problematic behavior in the society.
- The individual with high spiritual intelligence demonstrates higher measures of satisfaction and performance. Thus spiritual intelligence could be helpful in conflict management and peaceful co-existence in the society as it is a personal quality which enables the person to maintain both inner and outer peace and display love regardless of the circumstances whether stressed the individual is in or acute conflict.
- Substance use, school dropout and antisocial behaviour in adolescence lead to the decline in quality of life and mental health in adulthood. So the study may be implied to design health and wellness program in order to improve the resilience and mental health of adolescents.

- With respect to the cultivation of resilience among adolescents, one implication is that as adolescents develop toward adulthood, adverse situations will change as will their need for competencies. Therefore, a good person-stage-environment fit is required to keep pace with these changing needs and situations so that intervention programs remain developmentally appropriate to the target population.

- Furthermore, protective factors operate across different levels. In order for research to be realistic and interventions to be effective, we must consider how individual capacity interplays with external protective factors (skill, strength, resources, support or coping strategies). There is a need for more research on the interactions among adversities, internal and external protective factors, and interventions.

- Schools are a privileged avenue for the promotion of adolescent's positive development. In order to be effective in promoting adolescent's positive development, schools need to incorporate their objectives for the promotion of their healthy personality development.

- Family support can have a positive impact on adolescent's mental health by showing love, affection, care, showing interest in what is happening in child life, spending time together, encouraging the child and know his or her feeling, deal with the problem facing etc.

Limitation and Future Research Directions

In view of the limitation of the present study, the following suggestions may be made for further researches in the area.

- Sample taken for this study was not so large to generalize the findings although it provides a sense of insight for the future research.
- The role of the cultural factors has not been taken into account. Future researches must be based by adding cultural factor on these variables.
- The current study provides a cross-sectional snapshot of the relationship between spiritual intelligence, resilience, personality in relation to mental

health. Longitudinal data could be taken into account to validate the relationship between these variables.

- Sample taken for the study consisted of the adolescent's group. Further researches should focus on another sample to generalize the findings.
- The sample was taken only from different schools of Varanasi city situated in the Northern India carrying same organizational culture. More data could be included to generalize the finding on other parts of India having different organizational culture.
- Factor related to the school environment, teachers, and peer group could have been included in the study as they may be expected to play an important part in an adolescent's behaviour. Considering these factors, future research may result in better understanding of spiritual intelligence, resilience, personality and mental health in given population.
- The quantitative method of analyses has been used in the current study. Further research into the area may consider by employing qualitative methods to get a deeper insight into the mechanism of spiritual intelligence, resilience, personality and mental health.

CPSIA information can be obtained
at www.ICGtesting.com
Printed in the USA
LVHW040250020323
740706LV00017B/1630

9 782169 065144